# the complete
# pregnancy
# COOKBOOK

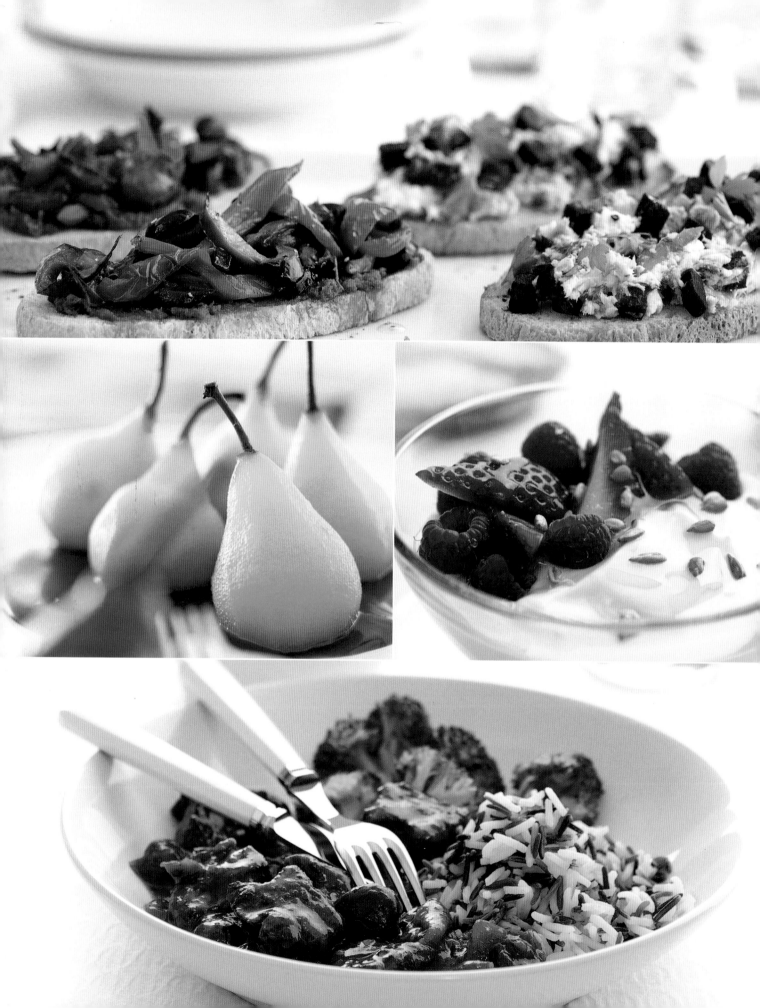

# the complete
# pregnancy
# COOKBOOK

**Fiona Wilcock**

MSc, PGCE, BA, RPHNutr

hamlyn

*This book is dedicated to my mother, Marie Smith,*
*who taught me so much about cooking and who died while*
*I was writing this edition.*

An Hachette UK Company
www.hachette.co.uk

First published in Great Britain in 2016 by Hamlyn,
a division of Octopus Publishing Group Ltd
Carmelite House, 50 Victoria Embankment
London EC4Y 0DZ
www.octopusbooks.co.uk

Distributed in the USA by Hachette Book Group
1290 Avenue of the Americas, 4th and 5th Floors
New York, NY 10020

Distributed in Canada by Canadian Manda Group
664 Annette St., Toronto, Ontario, Canada M6S 2C8

Text copyright © Fiona Wilcock 2016
Design and layout copyright © Octopus Publishing Group 2016

Art Director Chrissie Lloyd
Managing Art Editor Emily Breen
Photography Jules Selmes, David Murray
Home Economist Clare Lewis

ISBN 978 0 60063 220 7

1 3 5 7 9 10 8 6 4 2

Printed and bound in China

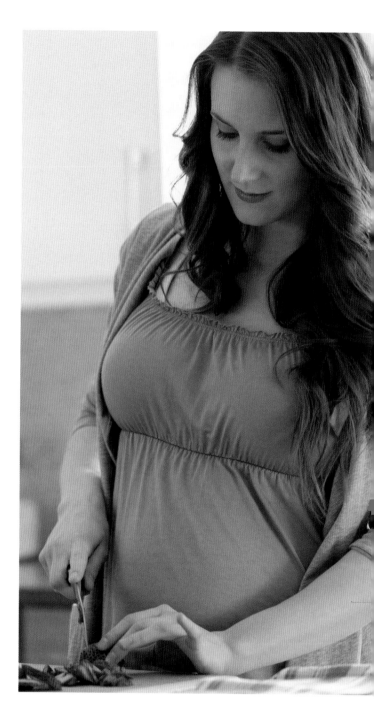

# CONTENTS

Introduction 6
How to use this book 7

### CHAPTER 1
## Eating Well 08

The key nutrients 10
Minerals 11
Vitamins 13
A healthy pregnancy diet 17

### CHAPTER 2
## Your Key Foods 18

Grains and potatoes 19
Glyemic index 19
Fruits 20
Vegetables 21
Herbs 22
Milk, cheese, and yogurt 22
Meat and poultry 24
Fish and shellfish 25
Eggs, legumes, and soy 25
Nuts and seeds 26
Water and other drinks 26
Fatty, sugary, and oily foods 27
Salty foods 27
Key supplements 27

### CHAPTER 3
## Looking After Yourself 28

Weight concerns 29
Making safe food choices 31
Food and common pregnancy
discomforts 36

### CHAPTER 4
## Menu Plans 38

About 39
First trimester 42
Second trimester 44
Third trimester 46
Newborn weeks 48

### CHAPTER 5
## Recipes 50

Breakfasts 51
Little bites, sandwiches, and salads 56
One-pot dishes 74
Poultry main dishes 84
Meat main dishes 96
Seafood main dishes 110
Vegetarian main dishes 120
Vegetables and side dishes 130
Desserts and baking 140

Nutritional analysis 154
Index 158
Acknowledgments 160

# INTRODUCTION

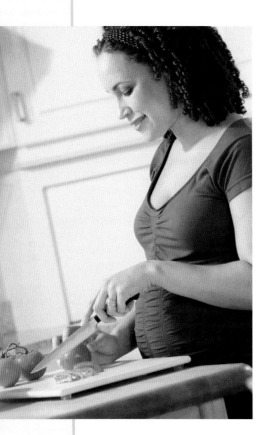

Pregnancy will be a very exciting time in your life, with a new person coming into being and growing inside you. It is also a time of huge emotional upheaval as you plan for the future, sometimes feeling anxious and worried, sometimes feeling euphoric, but there will be time for reflection as well, as you consider the moments that have passed, and look forward to a child-oriented life.

Pregnancy can also be a time of mixed health; you may feel overwhelmingly tired and have discomforts that you have never experienced, or you can look more lovely and feel sexier than you have ever done before.

Bound up with this whole physical and emotional experience is your diet. The nutrients you eat during pregnancy supply your baby with the essential building blocks for life and a have a significant effect on your child's long term health. Eating well is also vital in maintaining your own health and well-being, right from the time you think about having a baby through to after your baby is born. Food provides the nutrients and energy you'll need to get on with your everyday life—sometimes helping to ease common complaints—but it is also a source of pleasure as an occasional indulgent treat or a delicious dinner with family and friends.

The recipes in this book have been devised with all this in mind, and they contain the key nutrients you need to support pregnancy and breastfeeding. By checking the nutritional analysis pages, you'll easily be able to find recipes, which, for example, provide 25 percent or more of your daily needs for folic acid, iron, or vitamin C, even when cooking losses have been taken into account.

To make it even simpler, I've written and nutritionally analyzed weekly menu plans for each of the three trimesters and one for the newborn weeks. These allow for you to choose from a range of different recipes for breakfast, lunch, and dinner, and feel confident that your nutritional requirements will be met.

# HOW TO USE THIS BOOK

The Complete Pregnancy Cookbook provides you with the dietary information, meal plans, and recipes that will optimize both your nutrition and your enjoyment of food during your pregnancy.

Chapter One is about eating well in pregnancy, and you'll find this chapter particularly useful in understanding why you and your baby depend upon specific nutrients.

Chapter Two focuses on the foods that will help you achieve your pregnancy needs, providing plenty of suggestions and information on the different food groups.

Chapter Three is about feeling good in pregnancy, maintaining a healthy weight, making safe food choices, and using foods to deal with common pregnancy discomforts.

Chapter Four contains detailed menu plans that take you through the three trimesters to the early newborn weeks and breastfeeding. The recipe suggestions in italics are those that you can find in the book, but I also include easily prepared or store-bought dishes. The menu plans will make sure that you'll meet more than 90 percent of your requirements for all the major vitamins and minerals (*) throughout your pregnancy and while breastfeeding.

The RECIPES chapter contains more than 100 double-tested recipes designed to maximize your nutrition and to suit how you feel at various stages in your pregnancy. They are simple to make, allowing you to spend less time in the kitchen, and if you are not an experienced cook, there are simple instructions and tips to guide you. As well as substantial dishes for breakfast, lunch, and dinner, I've included a range of "little bites" for when you are not feeling that hungry and one-dish recipes for when you want to make as little mess in the kitchen as possible. Most of the recipes will serve two, but can often be doubled if you have visitors or are feeding other children, and many can be frozen. Each recipe contains preparation and cooking times and, if applicable, serving suggestions, storage, and allergy information.

Although the introduction will give you some idea of the essential nutrients each dish contains, there is a complete nutritional profile for each recipe at the back of the book.

*except vitamin D, which should be taken as a 400 IU supplement

### CHAPTER 1

# EATING WELL

This chapter explores what makes up a healthy pregnancy diet and how you can be sure you benefit from one. If you are already eating healthily, you may just have to make a few minor adjustments or, if you know that your diet really isn't as good as it should be, you will want to take a more critical look at what you eat. Increasingly we hear about the long-term consequences of eating well in pregnancy on a baby's future health (see box), so use this opportunity to find out more about a great diet, remembering it is never too early OR too late to improve the quality of what you eat.

## Not yet pregnant?

It is always best to plan ahead, so if you haven't yet conceived, being in good health will help. Trying to be the right weight for your height is a critical starting point (see page 29).

Apart from your prepregnancy weight, eating well before conceiving is important, because pregnancy places demands on your body's stores of many minerals and vitamins and may quickly deplete them. So an ideal prepregnancy diet is rich in key minerals, such as iron, calcium, iodine, magnesium, and zinc and important vitamins, especially folic acid and vitamin D. You can find out why these are important by looking at the later section in this chapter, and can make dishes, which are rich in these nutrients, by referring to the nutritional analysis of the recipes on page 154.

Because of their isoflavone content, which act like estrogens, soybeans can affect sperm concentrations; so if your partner normally consumes a lot of soy products, it may be a good idea for him to remove them from his diet while you are trying for a baby.

## Having twins or more?

Women carrying more than one baby require extra nutrients and additional calories to support the added increase in blood volume and uterine size as well as the development of two or more babies. In particular, this means an increased need for calcium, iron, and essential fatty acids, especially omega 3 fatty acids.

If you're having twins (or more babies), your diet needs to have a great mix of nutrient-rich foods. In addition to the 400 mcg of folic acid and 400 IU (10 mcg) of vitamin $D_3$ recommended for all pregnant women, you should talk to your healthcare provider about taking a prenatal supplement that provides zinc, magnesium, calcium, vitamin $B_6$, vitamin C, vitamin E, and iron. DHA (a fatty acid) is also important, so look for a supplement that contains 300 mg DHA without vitamin A (retinol).

## THE KEY NUTRIENTS

### Protein

Vital to every body cell, your baby needs you to eat protein-rich foods so that she can grow and develop normally. You also need protein to make the extra red blood cells required for your greatly increased blood volume.

Protein is made up of chains of amino acids—some of which your body can make while others must be found in foods. The latter are the essential amino acids, which are found almost exclusively in animal-base foods, such as meat, poultry, fish, and dairy products. Strict vegetarians, however, can be sure they have the right balance of amino acids by planning their diet carefully to include tofu and soy products as well as other beans, seeds, and grains.

### Carbohydrates

The main source of dietary energy, carbohydrates are easily broken down by the body to supply glucose. However, it's important to try to eat carbohydrate-rich foods that have been minimally processed, because these will be better at providing a more sustained release of glucose into the bloodstream instead of a peak followed by a low point, which may increase the risk of developing pregnancy diabetes. Put simply, it is a case of eating more whole-grain foods (and lower GI foods) and minimizing your use of sugars and sweetened drinks.

Good-quality carbohydrates are important, making a low carbohydrate, high protein diet unsuitable for women during pregnancy.

### Fats

The amount of fat in your diet should not increase in pregnancy, but you may need to pay attention to the quality of the fats you are eating to be sure your baby receives enough essential fatty acids. As with your prepregnancy diet, you should be keeping your intake of saturates down by using oils and spreads high in monounsaturates instead of saturates-rich butter, ghee, or animal-base spreads or frying fats. However, you do still need fat in your diet, so, in addition to oils, you should include nuts and seeds, which supply essential fatty acids, and avoid processed foods that supply partly hydrogenated (trans) fatty acids.

### Essential fatty acids

These are the fatty acids that the body can't generate itself so are needed in your diet. Commonly referred to as omega 3 fatty acids, alpha linolenic acid (ALA) is the most abundant in foods, and the body can convert this, to a limited degree, to DHA (docosahexanoic acid) and EPA (eicosapentaenoic acid). These are the two long chain omega 3 fatty acids that are vital for your baby's growth and development.

DHA is important because it plays a key role in the development and maturation of your baby's brain and eyes. The richest supply of DHA is oily fish, and one important project on maternal and infant nutrition recommended that all pregnant women should have a minimum of 200 mg of DHA a day, and eat fish at least once or twice a week, including oily fish, such as salmon, herring, and mackerel (see also page 32).

If you don't eat fish, you need to eat plenty of flaxseeds, omega 3 fortified eggs, and milk and green leafy vegetables. You can also look for specially formulated supplements of DHA/EPA designed for use in pregnancy.

### Fiber

There are two types, soluble and insoluble, and it's the latter's ability to keep things moving through your digestive system that is especially important during pregnancy.

Soluble fiber is broken down in the bowel and serves a number of bodily roles but in pregnancy, and it is its ability to help with satiety—keeping you feeling fuller—that can be useful if you are tempted to snack unhealthily. It is found in oats, peas, beans and lentils, and fruits, such as oranges, apples, and pears.

Insoluble fiber, because it is not broken down, helps prevent constipation by keeping waste moving through the digestive system. Constipation can be a particularly trying issue at this time, because pregnancy hormones affect the speed at which waste goes through your digestive tract. This type of fiber is found in whole-grain cereals, fruits, vegetables, and seeds.

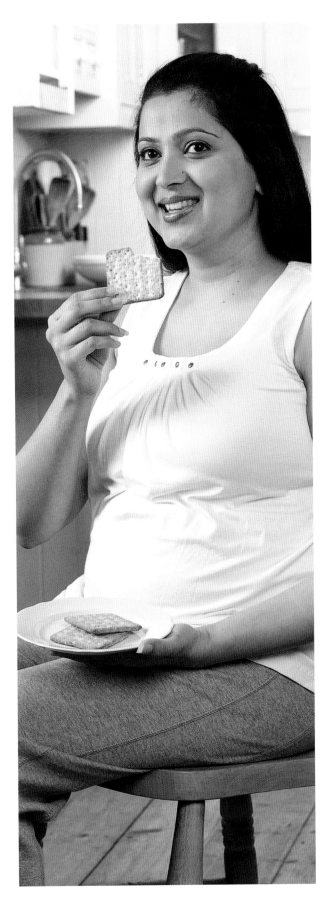

## MINERALS

### Calcium

It is essential for the proper growth and development of your baby's bones and teeth (your baby's first and adult teeth are developed by birth) as well as a healthy heart, muscles, and nervous system.

If you didn't eat calcium-rich foods before you became pregnant, your bone stores of calcium may be low, and this increases your risk of calcium deficiency. It is known that there is a link between poor calcium intake and preeclampsia—a serious medical condition that occurs only in pregnancy. However, calcium supplements of up to 1 g a day, can make sure that even women whose diet is low in calcium are less likely to have preeclampsia or preterm deliveries.

In the last trimester, your baby lays down a lot of bone and if you don't have adequate calcium in your diet, she will take it from your bones, leaving you more at risk of osteoporosis in later life. Your post pregnancy need for calcium also increases considerably when breastfeeding (see page 41).

Calcium works in conjunction with vitamin D (see page 16).

### Potassium and sodium

Both of these are essential for all-round health and are found in all body cells and fluids, including blood and lymph. Having the correct balance of fluids, especially in your blood, is crucial to your health. Salt is made up of sodium and another chemical called chloride. Too much sodium is known to increase your blood pressure, which increases your risk of high blood pressure (hypertension) in pregnancy.

One way of controlling your blood pressure is to increase the amount of potassium you eat. Potassium-rich foods include many fruits and vegetables and whole-grain cereals, so a healthy diet where you have a minimum of five portions of fruit and vegetables a day will certainly help provide plenty of it.

In the past, pregnant women were sometimes advised to limit their sodium intake to prevent the risk of preeclampsia, but there is little evidence that this is effective. However, if you regularly eat a lot of salty foods, cut down the amount of salt you use at the table and in cooking food before you become pregnant and don't increase it while you are pregnant.

## Magnesium

Another pregnancy essential, magnesium has a huge number of functions in your body, pregnant or not. These range from making protein and DNA for cells and tissues, ensuring the correct functioning of the nervous system to the more commonly understood role in bone formation. Magnesium is also involved in glucose and insulin metabolism, helping to make sure keep your blood sugar levels are kept constant.

Some medical conditions, such as cerebral palsy, sudden infant death syndrome, and mental retardation, may be linked to a magnesium deficiency, and many women, especially younger women, do not have enough magnesium.

Like calcium, magnesium is stored in your bones, so if your diet is poor for some time, you will start to deplete your stores. There is also some evidence that low levels of magnesium are linked to leg cramps and preeclampsia. Good sources include pumpkin, melon, and sunflower seeds; milk, bread, potatoes, and leafy green vegetables.

### Iron …

*Up to one in five women in the United States have inadequate iron in their diets. Therefore, about 20 percent of women probably enter pregnancy with low iron stores, and thus an increased risk of developing anemia. If you have heavy periods, don't eat iron-rich foods, such as meat, or have an ad hoc vegetarian diet, you are at greater risk of iron deficiency. Have a look at the recipes that provide iron (see page 154), and eat more of them or take a multivitamin and mineral supplement when you are planning a pregnancy.*

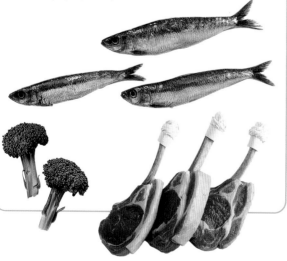

## Iron

Iron is essential for the manufacture of blood cells and your blood volume increases rapidly in pregnancy. Your growing placenta also uses iron, and it has been estimated that around 680 mg of iron is needed to meet your baby's growth need, which comes from any stored iron as well as your diet.

How much iron you need in pregnancy is hotly debated; in the UK, it is thought that because a pregnant woman has improved efficiency in absorbing iron from foods and is no longer losing blood each month, the requirements don't actually increase. In fact, the farther into pregnancy you go, the more efficient your body becomes at absorbing iron. However many women don't have enough iron in their diet while pregnant or before conceiving, meaning they probably don't have iron tucked away to call on when their needs increase. Women are more probable to have low iron stores if:

- The pregnancy is unplanned
- They've had a baby within the last eighteen months
- They don't eat red meat, such as beef or lamb, or other iron-rich foods
- They are still teenagers.

Having low iron stores increases your risk of developing iron deficiency anemia, and although your baby will preferentially take iron from you, there is more chance he will be born underweight.

Developing iron deficiency anemia in early pregnancy increases your risk of having a smaller placenta, which, in turn, can influence the size and health of your baby.

Becoming anemic in your second trimester can increase your risk of giving birth prematurely and also of having a low birth-weight baby. Recent studies have also found that by tracking populations now in their fifties, there is a link between iron deficiency anemia in the last trimester of pregnancy and schizophrenia in later life.

When breastfeeding, your milk supplies iron to your baby and your ability to absorb iron from food increases so that your baby get's enough iron. However, by around six months, breast milk alone does not meet your baby's need for iron.

## Zinc

Surveys show that many women do not have enough dietary zinc and are actually zinc deficient. It is also known that women who enter pregnancy with low zinc stores are at an increased risk of having a preterm baby. So it's important to consider this important nutrient when planning your diet, including zinc-rich sources, such as red meat, whole-grain cereals, beans, and lentils.

Preconceptually, zinc is also important for men, because it is an essential component of sperm.

Zinc and iron act antagonistically, so if you are prescribed iron supplements, you may need to increase your zinc intake, too, or take a multimineral supplemnt that provides both. As with calcium, your requirements only increase when you have had your baby and are breastfeeding, but unlike calcium, it can be harder to meet your requirements for zinc.

## Copper

The role of this little-known nutrient is becoming better established, and in pregnancy it seems to be important for your baby's brain development, particularly in the last few months of pregnancy. It also has a role in forming connective tissues in your baby's developing heart and immune system. Your need for copper does not increase in pregnancy, but if you are breastfeeding, you need to eat plenty of copper-rich foods, such as nuts, lentils, and shellfish.

## Selenium

This is an important antioxidant, which helps in many reactions in your body to protect you against cell damage, boosting your immune system in particular. As your body undergoes many complex changes during pregnancy, having adequate antioxidants is essential, and low levels of selenium in the diet have been associated with an increased risk of developing preeclampsia. The selenium content of a diet depends on the soil in which foods are grown and where animals graze. Good sources include fish, lentils, and sunflower seeds.

## Iodine

Iodine is vital because it is a component of the thyroid hormones that regulate your metabolism. A severe lack of iodine in the diet preconceptually and during pregnancy can lead to fetal brain damage, or cretinism, a developmental condition, which, thankfully is rare in developed countries.

In the United States, iodine deficiency is relatively uncommon because iodine is found in salt as well as dairy products and eggs. In addition fish, shellfish, and seaweeds contain it. However, women who avoid table salt, milk or milk products, and seafood, may not have enough dietary iodine. Vegan mothers-to-be, therefore, are recommended to have a daily supplement even if they are taking seaweed, because the amount varies (see also page 32). A supplement of 140 mcg started preconceptually and running throughout pregnancy would meet your needs.

## VITAMINS

### Vitamin A

Critical in pregnancy because it helps with the growth of all cells, vitamin A is essential for the development of your baby's organs, particularly eyes, and circulatory, respiratory, and nervous systems. Vitamin A is also important for your immune system, helping you fight disease and infection, as well as maintaining your vision. However, too much vitamin A can be dangerous, resulting in fetal malformations.

Vitamin A covers both retinol, which is found in animal foods, and carotenes, which are found in plant foods. The most commonly found carotene is beta carotene, which the body converts to retinol (the preferred source). Liver, which is a rich source of retinol, should not be eaten in pregnancy, nor should supplements that contain cod liver oil; these, too, contain too much retinol.

### Thiamin

Also known as vitamin $B_1$, it plays an important role in releasing energy from food; your requirements only increase in the last trimester and when you are breastfeeding. It is commonly found in peas, brown rice, and green vegetables and pork is an exceptionally good source.

## Riboflavin

Also known as vitamin $B_2$, it has a role in energy release, and your requirements increase throughout pregnancy and when breastfeeding.

Dairy foods are a great source of this vitamin, and many of the recipes provide it. If you don't eat dairy foods, consider a pregnancy dietary supplement and make sure you eat fortified foods, such as breakfast cereals or enriched soy drinks.

## Niacin

Also known as vitamin $B_3$, it is also important to help release energy from food, but additional quantities are not needed until you are breastfeeding. Like the other B vitamins, little is stored in the body, so it is important to have a regular dietary supply. Niacin is found in meat and fish, especially turkey, in cereals, and also in nuts.

Some studies have suggested that adequate niacin along with vitamins $B_6$ and $B_1$ can help prevent cleft palate and similar defects.

## Vitamin $B_6$

Also known as pyridoxine, it can be depleted with the long-term use of the contraceptive pill and is not readily stored in the body, so having a pregnancy diet rich in this nutrient is important. Pork, fish, whole grains, bread, eggs, and potatoes are good sources. Your baby needs it for the normal development of his central nervous system and brain. It is also an important antioxidant protecting your cells against damage and helping your immune defenses.

## Vitamin $B_{12}$

This plays a crucial role in making red blood cells and genetic material. Vitamin $B_{12}$ and folic acid both help convert a potentially harmful substance called homocysteine into a less harmful compound. This is important, because high levels of homocysteine in the body increase the risk of circulatory diseases and nervous system diseases that can affect you, and increase the risk of birth defects, especially neural tube defects, and result in premature birth and a low birth weight for your baby.

Vitamin $B_{12}$ is only found in animal foods or algae, meaning that strict vegetarians need to be sure of a supply from a supplement or fortified foods. Long-

term ovo-lacto vegetarians have been found to have lower levels of vitamin $B_{12}$ in their blood, which can predispose them to a deficiency in pregnancy, and a risk later on that their breast milk may supply inadequate amounts of $B_{12}$ to their babies.

## Folate

Or folic acid (the synthetic form) as it is more usually known to women, is an essential nutrient because it is well known to help reduce the risk of having a baby with neural tube defects (NTD). It also has other roles as described in vitamin $B_{12}$ above. Having a supplement of 400 mcg (micrograms) a day from before conception to the twelfth week of pregnancy is essential. If you previously had a baby with a neural tube defect, it should be increased to 4 mg and if you are diabetic, 5 mg. Insufficient folate in pregnancy can increase your risk of preterm delivery.

Folate in foods is susceptible to destruction, so it is important that food sources, of which the highest are vegetables, are carefully prepared and cooked to minimize loss.

Good sources are green leafy vegetables, especially Brussels sprouts and broccoli, asparagus, beet, oranges, whole grains, and black-eyed peas.

## Vitamin C

Perhaps the best known of the antioxidant vitamins, vitamin C, or ascorbic acid, plays an important role in protecting cells against damage, keeping your immune system working correctly, and in the proper development and functioning of the placenta. Ascorbic acid helps the digestive tract absorb iron from food, so is an essential part of a pregnancy diet, especially because only tiny quantities can be stored in the body.

Vitamin C is found in many fruits and vegetables but some can be lost through poor storage and cooking methods. Choose a quick cooking method

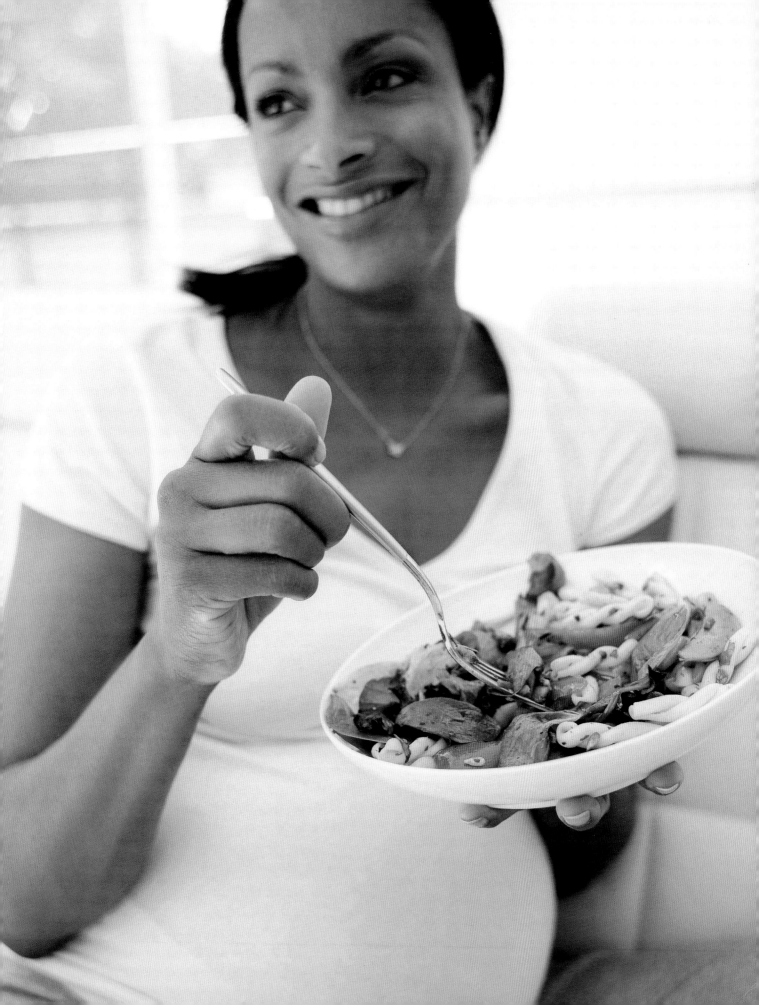

with minimum water, such as steaming or microwave cooking, and cut items into large pieces to minimize losses through oxidation.

## Vitamin D

It is essential for the body to effectively use calcium, and because it is found in few foods, milk, soy beverages and some orange juice and cereals are fortied. A daily supplement of 400 IU (10 mcg) may be recommended in pregnancy and breastfeeding. Actually, most vitamin D is made by the action of sunlight on skin, but you can't rely on sunshine to generate enough.

There are a number of reasons women go into pregnancy with low stores of vitamin D:

- Season: In the winter, due to lack of sun, we don't make any vitamin D.
- Latitude: The farther away from the equator you live, the less vitamin D you can make; for example, women living in Alaska have less chance to make it than women who live in Florida .
- Skin pigmentation: If you have black or dark skin, you make less than if you have white skin.
- Cultural practices: Eating a vegan diet or covering the skin to prevent exposure to sunlight will result in low levels.
- Blocking sun exposure: Using high-factor sunscreens to decrease the risk of skin cancer.

If you become pregnant with low levels of stored vitamin D and don't take supplements, it may increase your risk of developing preeclampsia and pregnancy diabetes. There is also the possibility of longer term consequences, such your baby's bones being poorly mineralized in early childhood, which in turn leads to rickets. There is also some evidence that persistent wheezing in childhood may be linked to poor vitamin D status in pregnancy. Obviously, adequate vitamin D while breastfeeding helps to make sure your baby's bones can form properly, and that when he starts to walk, they are strong enough to support him and ward off rickets.

## Vitamin E

A group of compounds called tocopherols form Vitamin E, and they are important protective antioxidants. There is some evidence that low intakes of vitamin E are linked to an increased risk of preeclampsia. Vitamin E is widely distributed in foods, and is carried into the body like other fat soluble vitamins in dietary fats and oils. During pregnancy you should be getting 15 mg (22.5 IU) a day and the amount increases to 19 mg (28.5 IU) when breastfeeding.

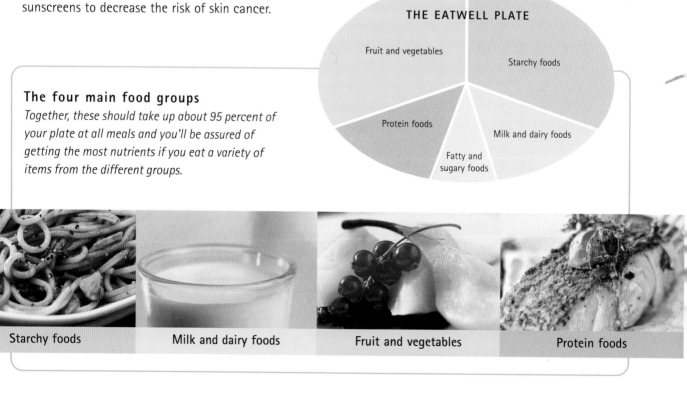

**THE EATWELL PLATE**

Fruit and vegetables

Starchy foods

Protein foods

Milk and dairy foods

Fatty and sugary foods

### The four main food groups

*Together, these should take up about 95 percent of your plate at all meals and you'll be assured of getting the most nutrients if you eat a variety of items from the different groups.*

Starchy foods

Milk and dairy foods

Fruit and vegetables

Protein foods

## Vitamin K

This fat soluble vitamin is essential for blood clotting and routinely given to newborn babies to prevent a rare hemorrhaging disease. There are no specific recommendations for this in pregnancy or breastfeeding, and making sure that you eat green vegetables will provide a good supply.

## A HEALTHY PREGNANCY DIET

### The four main food groups

Whether pregnant or not, a balanced diet comprises eating a mixture of foods from four of the food groups illustrated by the "Eatwell plate." Each of these groups contains a wide range of foods that supply a host of different nutrients, and you should aim to eat the relative proportions of them, which the plate suggests. There is a fifth group, which are the foods high in fat and sugar. these should to be eaten in only limited amounts, because they supply few valuable nutrients, but the tend to be the easiest ones in which to over indulge. See below.

### Starchy foods

Bread, rice, potatoes, pasta, and cereals are among the foods rich in carbohydrates, which supply energy and the B group vitamins. Make sure that at every meal you fill at least one-third of your plate with these types of foods. Choose whole-grain versions or brown rice for additional fiber and other nutritional benefits. Look for fortified bread and breakfast cereals.

### Fruits and vegetables

Whether fresh, frozen, dried, or canned (in water or juice), these contain a wide range of vitamins, minerals, and phytochemicals essential for a healthy pregnancy. Make sure you have a minimum of five portions every day (not counting potatoes), which should cover between one-third and half your plate, and eat a variety of different colors and types to obtain all the different nutrients and protective substances. Keep in mind that fruit or vegetable juices count as only one portion.

### Milk and dairy foods

As well as milk, yogurt, and cheese, this group includes vegetarian sources, such as soy milk and "yogurts." (Butter, cream, and eggs are not dairy foods). These foods provide protein as well as calcium and the B group vitamins, especially $B_{12}$ and $B_2$. Make sure you have three portions or the equivalent a day and choose reduced fat versions, because they provide less fat, calories, and saturates. If you can't or don't eat dairy foods, have calcium from other sources. Fortified soy milk and yogurts are a great alternative, and canned fish, such as sardines, contain a lot of calcium if you eat the bones.

### Protein-rich foods

Meat, poultry, fish, eggs, beans, lentils, and nuts are major sources of protein, as well as supplying key minerals, such as iron, zinc, and magnesium (see details on page 11). Fish contain iodine and oily fish omega 3 fatty acids (see page 24) and lentils, chickpeas, beans, seeds, and nuts contain zinc, calcium, magnesium, selenium, and iron.

Eat a high protein source at two meals a day. If you don't eat meat, poultry, or fish, make sure you eat legumes, tofu, and textured soy protein as well as eggs and cheese to obtain dietary essentials without having too many saturates.

### Fatty and sugary foods and beverages

Cookies, cakes, potato chips, ice creams, carbonated drinks, chocolate, etc., offer variety, interest, and palatability to your diet, but they are really extras not essentials. They are especially energy dense—that is, they contain high levels of fat and sugar in a small volume and usually provide few useful vitamins and minerals.

Oils, whether olive, canola, corn, or sunflower, are around 99 percent pure fat and while they provide some fatty acids the body can convert to omega 3 fatty acids, be careful not to have too much.

Many types of butter and fat spreads are available with reduced levels of fat, saturates, and calories, so choose these over the normal versions. Use spreads rich in monounsaturates, such as olive spread.

### CHAPTER 2

# YOUR KEY FOODS

This chapter looks at individual foods and food groupings to highlight their specific nutrient value and provide guidelines on what and how much to eat, as well as gives you advice on any special care that you need to be taking.

## Grains and potatoes

These two items and the products made from them, such as pasta, bread, and some breakfast cereals, are a healthy source of energy, because they are high in carbohydrates and usually low in fat. They should provide between 45 and 60 percent of the energy (calories) you eat. Low carbohydrate diets that limit this food group are not suitable during pregnancy.

The quality of the carbohydrate you eat is important, and eating whole-grain or brown types of pasta, bread, cereals, or grains are a better choice because more nutrients are provided.

"Whole grain" refers to the grain after the removal of inedible parts but must include the entire germ, endosperm, and bran. Whole grains include brown and wild rice, whole wheat flour, and products made from it, such as bread and pasta, and whole grains of pot barley, corn, millet, buckwheat, rye, and quinoa. Pot barley sold in health food stores has the husk partly or completely removed. Look for the higher fiber brown grains instead of the polished white ones.

### Did you know?
*Because Westerners eat plenty of potatoes, they make a great contribution to our vitamin C intake. New potatoes contain the most.*

### Fiber in breakfast cereals

| Product | Average portion size | Fiber content g |
|---|---|---|
| All Bran | 6 tablespoons | 10.3 |
| Oatmeal, homemade | 1 bowl | 1.3 |
| Shredded Wheat cereal | 2 big biscuits | 4.4 |
| Cornflakes | 5 tablespoons | 0.3 |
| Unsweetened muesli | 3 tablespoons | 3.4 |

Apart from energy and fiber, whole grains are good sources of the B group vitamins, zinc, and iron.

This food group, too, is a great source of fiber, and apart from preventing constipation in pregnancy, fiber can help keep pregnancy blood sugars more even and reduce the risk of other pregnancy complications, including preeclampsia.

There is no extra requirement for fiber in pregnancy, but getting the minimum of 25 g per day can be difficult, and most Americans take in only 15 g a day. Eating whole grains or whole wheat versions where possible can make a huge impact. The fiber content of some typical breakfast cereals are listed above.

Another measure of carbohydrate quality is the glycemic index. Studies indicate that the risk of pregnancy diabetes increases if you eat high GI foods (see below).

## Glycemic index

This measures how a particular food affects your blood glucose when you eat it. The lower the GI, the better. A low GI means the carbohydrate is released slowly so that you stay feeling fuller for longer, and your body doesn't have a rush of blood sugar followed by a slump.

Studies have shown that mothers-to-be who eat high GI foods, which are released more quickly, will probably have high sugar levels in pregnancy and pregnancy complications. If you have pregnancy diabetes, you should eat low GI foods, because these will help to keep your blood sugar under better control. The table below shows you how to choose lower GI foods.

## GI of starchy carbohydrate foods

0-55 is low

56-69 is moderate

70 and over is high

| Food | Glycemic index |
| --- | --- |
| White bread | 70 |
| Whole wheat bread | 69 |
| Stoneground whole meal bread | 53 |
| Rye bread | 50 |
| White boiled rice | 98 |
| White boiled basmati rice | 58 |
| Brown rice | 68 |
| Whole wheat pasta e.g spaghetti | 37 |
| White pasta e.g spaghetti | 41 |
| Udon noodles | 62 |
| Pearl barley | 25 |
| Oatmeal with water | 42 |
| Potatoes, new boiled | 62 |
| Potatoes, boiled | 56 |
| Potatoes, mashed | 70 |
| Potatoes, baked | 85 |
| Couscous | 65 |
| Quinoa | 53 |
| Bulgur (cracked wheat) | 46 |
| All Bran | 38 |
| Cornflakes | 93 |
| Muesli | 56 |
| Wheat biscuit cereal | 69 |
| Rye crackers | 64 |

## Fruits

The choice is almost endless these days because new varieties appear frequently in our markets. Try to eat seasonally when you can, not forgetting favorites such as oranges, nectarines, plums, apples, and pears.

Fruit is a pregnancy essential because it provides a wide variety of different vitamins, minerals, and protective plant nutrients (phytochemicals). A great source of vitamin C (for the maximum amount, eating ripe fruit raw and in season is about as good as it gets) and sometimes betacarotene, fruits also provide essential dietary fiber. One of the reasons that fruit juice only counts once in your five a day is that it contains almost no fiber, so make sure you have whole fruit as well as juice.

Many of the phytochemicals found in fruits (and other plant foods) act as antioxidants and prevent cells from being damaged. There are many thousands of these and because some are only just being identified, researchers have not yet pinpointed those that may be of special benefit in pregnancy. However, the benefits of having plenty of whole fruits in the diet is well known.

- Red grapes and cranberries contain resveratrol, which is not only thought to slow the aging process, but it has anti-inflammatory properties that are great at any stage of life.
- Apples and berries contain quercetin, another protective antioxidant
- Strawberries are not only a rich source of vitamin C, but also provide folate, and a protective antioxidant, ellagic acid.
- Papaya contains large quantities of both vitamin C and betacarotene.
- Many fruits contain potassium, which is important in regulating blood pressure, and the much-derided prune, or dried plum, is an excellent source.
- Melon, especially cantaloupe is packed with betacarotene.
- Bioflavonoids of which grapefruit are a particularly rich source may help reduce water retention and swelling in the legs, a common pregnancy problem.
- Red and purple berries contain antioxidants called anthocynanins, which are thought to help reduce the risk of developing cancers and heart disease by protecting cells from damage.

## Nutritional benefits of different fruits

| Item | Average portion | Approx. calories | Why it's a great pregnancy snack |
| --- | --- | --- | --- |
| Apple | 1 medium | 46 | Few calories, filling, thirst quenching, cheap, provides fiber, low GI |
| Apricots (dried) | 3 medium | 75 | Rich source of fiber; source of iron, and betacarotene. Easy to store |
| Bananas | 1 medium | 95 | Easy to eat and digest, provides fiber and potassium, medium GI |
| Blueberries | 2 handfuls | 50 | Great antioxidant protection |
| Kiwifruit | 2 fruit | 40 | Rich source of vitamin C, and potassium |
| Oranges | 1 medium | 45 | Rich source vitamin C. Source of folate and low GI |
| Peaches | 1 medium | 36 | Source of vitamin C, thirst quenching, cheap in season |
| Pears | 1 medium | 51 | Source of fiber, cheap in season |
| Pineapple | 1 large slice | 33 | Source of vitamin C, thirst quenching, |
| Plums | 2 medium | 28 | Cheap in season, source betacarotene and fiber |
| Prunes (dried plums) | 3 medium | 56 | Rich in fiber, potassium, contains iron. Easy to store |
| Strawberries | 7 strawberries | 27 | Rich source of vitamin C, and antioxidants. Best when in season |

## Vegetables

These also come in different colors—green, purple, white, orange, and red—and the differently colored ones contain a variety of vitamins, minerals, and phytochemicals, which are essential for you and your growing baby. Eating five portions of vegetables a day as well as a fruit or glass of fruit juice will help you get a daily supply of baby building essentials.

Carrots and other orange colored vegetables, such as sweet potatoes and squash, supply carotenoids, a form of betacarotene and vitamin A. Surprisingly, so do dark green veggies, such as kale and spinach. Not only does vitamin A protect you by boosting immunity, it is essential for your baby's development, especially that of her lungs.

Many vegetables are rich in folate, too. Asparagus, beet, chicory, spinach leaves, Swiss chard, baby corn, and Brussels sprouts all contain more than 80 mcg of folate per 2¾ ounce portion. If cooking, steam them lightly to preserve as much of this heat sensitive vitamin as possible.

Green leafy vegetables are a great source of magnesium, which you and your baby need. Magnesium is at the heart of the green plant pigment chlorophyll, so if it's green you'll be getting some.

### All the colors of the rainbow

*Fruits come in different colors and each signals different nutrients and phytochemicals. Make sure you eat from across the range.*

**Red** *strawberries, red grapes, red apples, raspberries, rhubarb, plums, red currants, red grapefruit.*

**Green** *kiwifruit, green grapes, green apples, avocado.*

**Yellow** *pears, pineapples, some melons.*

**Purple** *blueberries, plums, cherries, blackberries, black currants.*

**Orange** *clementines and satsumas, apricots, melons, persimmon, mango, papaya, nectarines, and peaches.*

vegetables

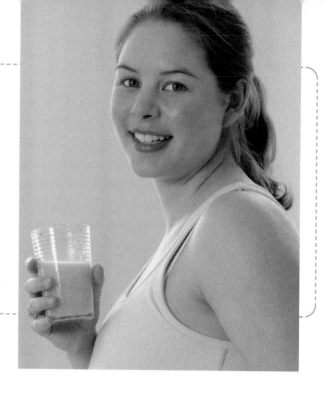

### Did you know?

*Some vegetables provide iron, but it is less well absorbed by the body than the iron found in meat or other animal foods. However, to make sure you absorb as much as possible, avoid drinking tea or coffee at meal times, and have a vitamin C rich food at the same meal. A glass of unsweetened citrus juice, a few cherry tomatoes, a kiwifruit, or a bowl of seasonal strawberries are all great candidates.*

Seaweed is a good source of iodine. However, brown seaweeds (kelp, kombu, wakame, quandai-cai, hiziki/hijiki, arame, or Sargassum fusiforme), which are usually sold for stews, contain so much you could overdose on the iodine, which could adversely effect your baby's health. Choose the lower iodine containing red or green seaweeds, which are sold for sushi (e.g Nori) instead.

### Herbs

Although the green part of plants used to flavor or season a dish are unlikely to have any medicinal benefit (due to the small amount normally used), herbs can add small quantities of vitamins, minerals, and phytochemicals. Parsley is a great source of vitamin C, for example, but you would have to munch through a $1\frac{1}{2}$ ounce bunch to have the same amount as eating one orange. Wash any herbs before use, making sure they do not have any soil left on them.

### Milk, cheese, and yogurt

Known for their contribution to calcium intakes, milk, yogurt, and cheese have other baby building credentials, such as protein, iodine, vitamin $B_2$ (riboflavin), and $B_{12}$ (cyanocobalamin). If you don't or can't eat this food group, it is really important to be sure that you are getting equivalent nutrition from alternative foods (see box, page 23). Substituting soy products for milk and yogurt is great, but make sure that they are fortified, especially if you don't eat meat as well (see also page 24).

Aim to have at least three portions of dairy products or equivalent a day. For about two-thirds

**BE CAREFUL**

*Some unpasteurized, mold ripened or blue varieties of cheese carry a risk of listeriosis, which can have serios pregnancy complications (see also page 31).*

### Calcium-rich recipes

- *Stuffed Portobello Mushrooms*
- *Sardine and Red Pepper Strudel*
- *Egg, Tomato, and Onion Roll*
- *Cheddar and Sun-Dried Tomato Biscuits*

of your 1,000 mg calcium requirement try one of these combinations:

- 1 (8 fluid ounce) glass lowfat milk + $\frac{1}{2}$ cup low fat yogurt + 1 ounce piece hard cheese *or*
- 1 (8 fluid ounce) glass fortified soy milk + 1 large canned sardine with bones *or*
- $3\frac{1}{2}$ oz tofu + 1 tablespoon sesame seeds + 2 dried figs.

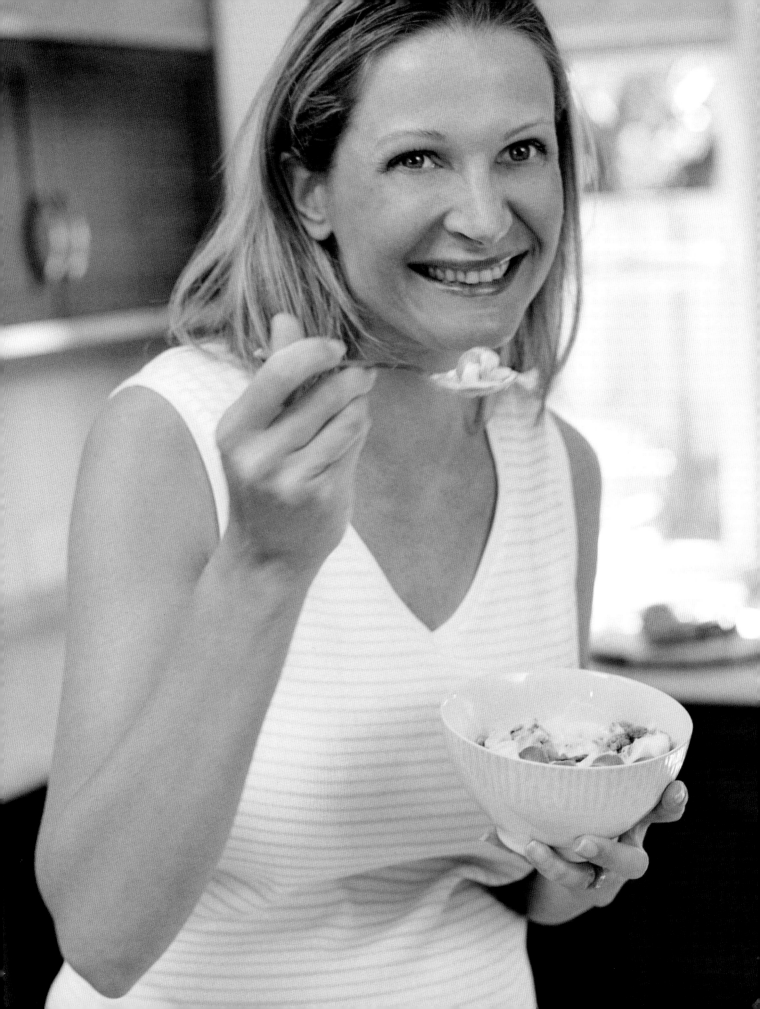

## Meat and poultry

Although these foods are known for their high protein content, they are packed with other important vitamins and minerals, which your body absorbs easily, especially during pregnancy.

Meats and poultry are, in general, great sources of iron, zinc, and vitamin $B_{12}$, but some provide a particularly rich source of certain nutrients. For example, pork for thiamin ($B_1$), beef for iron, turkey for zinc and niacin, and lamb and beef for vitamin $B_{12}$. However, liver and any liver products, such as paté or paste, should be avoided, because they can have unhealthily high levels of retinol (vitamin A).

### Did you know?

*Duck contains more healthy monounsaturated fat than saturated fat. By broiling or dry frying a duck breast and removing the skin, you will consume less than 200 calories yet receive around half of your pregnancy needs for zinc, and more than one-third for iron. If you include the skin, the amount of fat obviously increases, but so does the flavor! Perhaps make it an occasional treat?*

### Pro- and prebiotics in pregnancy

*Probiotic (cultures containing "good" bacteria) mini yogurt based drinks are frequently consumed and are safe in pregnancy—just make sure you follow the use-by dates. A few studies have looked at whether probiotics may actually improve the health of pregnant women and one found that women who took probiotic supplements were less likely to develop pregnancy diabetes. However, further studies need to be carried out to confirm this as well as discover if prebiotics (substances often naturally found in certain items, such as leeks and bananas, on which "good" digestive bacteria may grow) have other benefits to mother and her growing baby.*

### Calcium rich alternatives

*Calcium is an essential mineral in pregnancy and when nursing so be sure you have some of these calcium rich alternatives if you don't have milk, yogurt, or cheese regularly.*

- *Tofu*
- *Sardines or other canned fish with bones*
- *Fortified soy milk or yogurt*
- *Baked beans*
- *Curly kale or spinach*
- *Figs, especially dried or ready to eat*

Meat has had a lot of negative press over the last few years with concerns about its link to cancer and its saturates content. While there are issues with consuming a lot of processed meats such as frankfurters, salamis, and poor quality hamburgers, eating lean red meat with all visible fat removed a couple of times a week does not pose a danger. Indeed, the zinc, iron, and vitamin $B_{12}$, which are provided and readily absorbed from meat, supply dietary essentials. Whether you are planning a pregnancy or already pregnant, unless for religious or ethical reasons you can't or don't eat meat, do try to include lean meat in your diet at least once a week.

## Fish and shellfish

Another great source of protein, fish also provide iodine and, to a lesser or greater degree, depending on the variety, the long chain fatty acids known as omega 3. Some fish are also rich in vitamins A and D. However, some fish contain unacceptable levels of mercury and/or other chemicals (see page 32).

Fish are grouped into two major types: white and oily. White fish, such as halibut, cod, coley, pollack, red snapper, tilapia, sole, flounder, dab, etc., are safe

to eat in pregnancy and are very low in fat but contain very little omega 3.

Oily fish, such as trout, salmon, herring, mackerel, sardines, pilchards, anchovies, and sprats, are safe to eat in pregnancy and are a great source of omega 3 fatty acids and provide essential vitamins A and D.

Shellfish, such as mussels, shrimp, crab, lobster, crayfish, and squid, are safe to eat in pregnancy when cooked. They all contain, iodine, selenium, and copper and mussels, squid, and crab contain omega 3. Avoid oysters, because they are usually eaten raw.

## Eggs, legumes, and soy products

These foods are great for nonmeat eaters, supplying a range of different types of nutrients. Each has its own benefits, so try to eat a little of them all.

Make sure you keep your eggs refrigerated, use them by their expiration date, and cook them thoroughly to reduce the risk of food poisoning from bacteria.

Legumes are beans, peas, and lentils and are a cheap supply of protein as well as the B group vitamins, iron, and zinc. Black-eyed peas are unusually high in folate: three tablespoons provide 60 percent of your daily requirement. Lentils and most beans provide at least 2 mg of iron per ½ cup portion.

Soybeans are an amazingly versatile food and the only bean that contains all eight essential amino acids, making it of equal to the protein of animal foods. The boiled beans are a good source of iron, folate, biotin, and provide dietary fiber. Tofu or bean

### Easy ways with fish

- *Mash one canned sardine with lemon juice and spread on whole wheat toast, broil until hot.*
- *Microwave a skinless salmon fillet and while it is cooking stir fry two chopped scallions, slices of red bell pepper and snow peas, and a handful of bean sprouts. Stir in a sauce made with 1 teaspoon grated ginger, garlic, splash of sherry, and 1 teaspoon reduced sodium soy sauce. Serve with whole wheat or udon noodles.*
- *Place a white fish fillet on a few fine asparagus spears, top with chopped marinated artichokes, grated lemon zest, a squirt of lemon juice, and bake for 20 minutes.*
- *Heat one tablespoon of canola oil in a saucepan and quickly cook a large handful of raw shrimp and a clove of crushed garlic until the shrimp are pink. Serve on top of a bed of leaves with a multigrain roll for a quick lunch.*

### Nutritional content of eggs

| Nutrient | Amount in one egg | % of pregnancy requirement |
| --- | --- | --- |
| Vitamin A mcg | 98 | 16 |
| Vitamin D mcg | 0.9 | 9 |
| Vitamin $B_2$ mcg | 0.24 | 22 |
| Vitamin $B_{12}$ mcg | 1.3 | 86 |
| Iodine mcg | 27 | 19 |
| Selenium mcg | 6 | 10 |

curd is a rich source of calcium, and also contains some iron.

If you are a vegan, beware of having too many soy products, because they contains factors that can interfere with your body's ability to absorb and use iodine.

## Nuts and seeds

These are a great source of vitamin E, and also the shorter omega 3 fatty acids, which the body can convert to long chain omega 3 fatty acids. Some are a great source of individual nutrients, but normally you only eat only small amounts. The following are "superrich" in various nutrients:

- Sesame seeds in calcium, iron, magnesium, and copper.
- Pumpkin seeds in iron, magnesium, and zinc.
- Sunflower seeds in magnesium, and vitamin E.
- Flaxseed (linseed) in zinc and magnesium.
- Brazil nuts in selenium and vitamin E.
- Almonds in biotin (they also contain calcium).
- Hazelnuts in biotin and vitamin E.
- Peanuts in vitamin E and biotin.

Seeds are a key supply of magnesium, an important pregnancy mineral, so nibbling on them can boost your supply.

## Water and other drinks

Being hydrated in pregnancy is crucial and even more so when you are breastfeeding. I even devoted an entire book, *Super Drinks for Pregnancy,* to the subject. It contains dozens of recipes accompanied by full nutritional analyzes.

Mothers-to-be should drink around 9¾ cups of fluids a day and breastfeeding mothers 10–11 cups. It is expected that 70–80 percent of this fluid will come from drinks including water, and the remainder from water-containing foods (especially vegetables and fruit).

Fluids can be water or watery drinks, such as herbal and fruit teas, milk or milky drinks, and fruit juices or smoothies. However, you will want to limit your intake of caffeine containing drinks, such as green and black teas and coffee, because more than 200 mg caffeine per day is not recommended (see page 35).

Carbonated flavored drinks, even diet versions, provide few nutrients, and it would be better to drink a glass of milk or water—both for your teeth and the

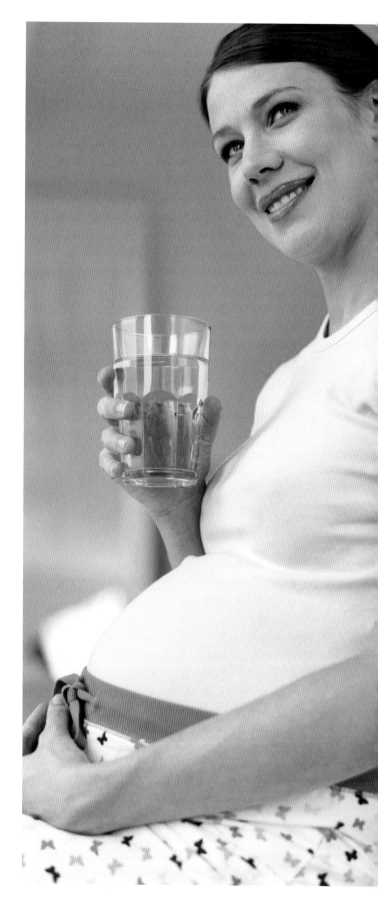

nutrition your baby receives. It is also very easy to overconsume calories by drinking sweetened beverages, and drinking large amounts could increase your risk of having pregnancy diabetes. So limit the number of sugary drinks you have. One glass of fruit juice or a smoothie a day is enough.

## Fatty, sugary, and oily foods

No one could argue that cakes, cookies, ice cream, or chocolates are pregnancy essentials, even though cravings can make them seem so. They add very little to your diet and may displace healthier foods, so limit the amount you eat. If you do eat them, choose small portions, and first have some milk and/or a piece of fruit. This way you will obtain vital nutrients and have less space for the less nutritious treat.

Oils and dressings are usually high in fat, so limit these, using oils high in monounsaturated fatty acids such as olive or canola oil. Try balsamic glaze or a spritz of lemon juice on your salad, or choose the lowest fat mayonnaise or mix some with fat-free yogurt. Butter is high in saturates, so either replace it with a mono- or polyunsaturated spread, preferably reduced in fat, or use a reduced fat butter if you can't give up the taste.

All sugars, syrups, and honey are similar in their energy value. Try to have as little as possible, being even more strict if you have pregnancy diabetes. Use one of the many sugar substitutes now available; all are safe in pregnancy. Xylitol is included in some of the recipes.

## Salty foods

Most condiments are fine to eat in pregnancy but be careful with sodium. Most people far exceed the daily 2,300 mg recommendation. Be careful not to have too many snacks, such as salted nuts, pickles, olives,

sausages, bacon, salami, and other preserved meats. Many everyday foods that are also high in sodium include breads, cheeses, prepared meals, and soups.

## Key supplements

Apart from the 400 mcg of folic acid you need from before you conceive until the twelfth week of pregnancy, make sure you also take a supplement with 400 IU of vitamin D. These two vitamin supplements are pregnancy essentials that are not easily obtained in the required amounts from foods.

If you want to take an all-round supplement, ask your healthcare provide to recommend a pregnancy supplement that have been formulated to take into account your increased nutrient requirements using safe levels of vitamins and minerals. Some also supply essential omega 3 fatty acids. Do not use cod liver oil or other fish oil supplements if they contain vitamin A as retinol.

Strict vegetarians are advised to carefully plan their diet, and an comprehensive multivitamin and mineral supplement is recommended.

**Best for folate**
*One 3 ounce portion of the following contains more than 80 mcg of folate. Steam lightly to preserve as much of this heat sensitive vitamin as possible.*

- *Asparagus, steamed*
- *Beet, boiled or roasted*
- *Purple sprouting broccoli*
- *Chicory, raw*
- *Spinach leaves, raw*
- *Swiss chard, boiled*
- *Baby corn, boiled*
- *Brussel sprouts boiled*

### CHAPTER 3

# LOOKING AFTER YOURSELF

Food supplies you with the vital nutrients necessary to maintain a pregnancy and support your baby's growth, so it's important to know which ones to avoid and how to prepare food safely. Managing your weight also has a great impact on the health of you and your baby.

## WEIGHT CONCERNS

Being the "right" weight when you conceive will give your baby a great start in life, but many pregnancies are unplanned, so you may need to make adjustments. Being pregnant does not give you a green light to eat for two. The more unnecessary weight you gain, the harder it is to lose afterward, and your baby needs a healthy active mom at all times. If you are overweight at the start of your pregnancy, it's really important to manage your weight. The greater your weight, especially with a BMI >30, the greater the risk of:

- Having a baby with birth defects (e.g. spina bifida or cleft lip or palate)
- Miscarriage or still birth
- Preeclampsia;
- Pregnancy diabetes
- Complications in labor, including having a Caesarean section.

Being very overweight can also increase your baby's risk of long-term health problems. It is now believed that what happens to your baby while you are carrying her can influence the way she responds to a host of factors after birth and into later life. Looking after yourself in pregnancy and eating a healthy diet, along with avoiding gaining too much weight, is important to minimize the effect of this "metabolic programming."

Overly thin moms to be tend to have underweight babies and are more at risk of miscarriage. Women who have a BMI of 18.5 or less often find it difficult to conceive, and they may be advised to gain some weight before trying to get pregnant. If you are underweight because you restrict your diet in any way—whether you have an eating disorder, eschew certain food groups, or are particularly choosy—it is really important to deal with these issues before you become pregnant. Your baby needs a constant supply of nutrients and relies on you eating a healthy balanced diet to provide a wide range of vitamins, minerals, and, crucially, energy from carbohydrates, fat, and protein. Dieting and binging are off-limits in pregnancy.

### How much weight should I gain?

You obviously need to make sure you are eating enough, but how much is that really when, after your baby is born, you don't want to have to worry about months of hard work to get your figure back.

The best way to tell if you are a healthy weight is to work out your body mass index (BMI). To do so, divide your weight in pounds by your height in inches squared and multiply by 703. (For example, if you are 5 feet 6 inches and weigh 146 pounds, the calculation is: 5 x 12 = 60, then 60 + 6 = 66 inches; 66 x 66 = 4,356; 146 ÷ 4,356 = 0.0335; 0.0335 x 703 = 23.56. Once you are pregnant, the U.S. Institute of Medicine guidelines (2009) provide a useful guide for weight gain based on your prepregnancy weight (see page 30). You will be weighed and your abdomen measured at each prenatal checkup.YYour energy

### Measuring weight
*Although it has some limitations, many health professionals use body mass index (BMI) to assess weight. The ranges below apply to healthy adults.*

| | |
|---|---|
| *less than 20* | *underweight* |
| *20–25* | *healthy* |
| *25–30* | *overweight* |
| *Over 30* | *obese* |

## Weight gain for singleton pregnancy

| Prepregnancy weight status | BMI | Recommended gain in pounds |
|---|---|---|
| Underweight | <18.5 | 28–40 |
| Healthy weight | 18.5–24.9 | 25–35 |
| Overweight | 25.0–29.9 | 15–25 |
| Obese | >30.0 | 11–20 |

## Weight gain for twin+ pregnancy

| Prepregnancy weight status | BMI | Recommended gain in pounds |
|---|---|---|
| Normal | 18.5–24.9 | 37–54 |
| Overweight | 25–29.9 | 31–50 |
| Obese | >30 | 25–42 |

### Your energy needs

Like most moms, you may be somewhat surprised to discover that you really don't need to eat more for the first two trimesters. Your body is amazing at utilizing what you eat as well as your body stores to supply your baby with many of her needs. Throughout pregnancy, different hormones are used to mobilize your stores of fat and nutrients, and your digestive system becomes increasing efficient at absorbing nutrients from foods. This, coupled with a decrease

### Where does the weight go?

*You can expect to gain an average of 30 pounds throughout your pregnancy, and here is where the weight goes.*

| | |
|---|---|
| *Breast and uterus enlargement* | *3 pounds* |
| *Placenta* | *2 pounds* |
| *Baby* | *7–8 pounds* |
| *Amniotic fluid* | *2 pounds* |
| *Additional blood and fluids* | *7 pounds* |
| *Fat deposits for breastfeeding* | *8 pounds* |

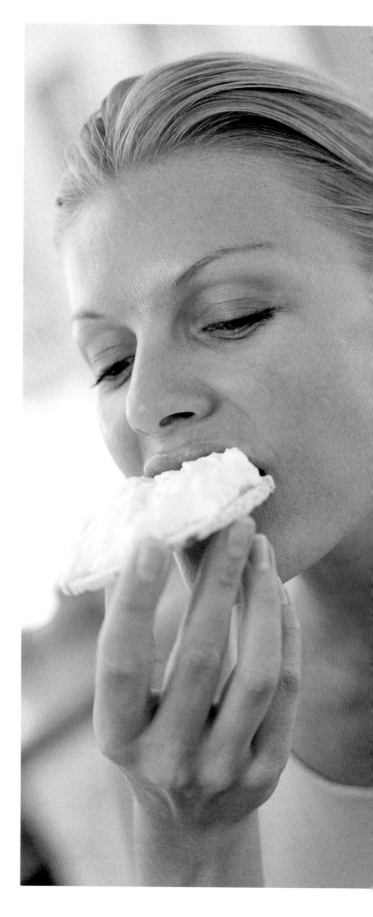

## Stay active

*Being physically active is a great way to help manage your weight even when pregnant; it can also help your body prepare for labor, increase your stamina, and keep you supple. Most women are able to carry out some exercise, whether it is simply walking, doing housework or gardening, or carrying on with a routine at the gym or swimming pool. Activity of any kind can also help control your blood sugar levels, which may reduce your risk of developing pregnancy diabetes.*

*Your body adapts to exercise during pregnancy, and this seems to protect your baby from potential harm, so not only is doing some gentle exercise good for you and your baby now, it can help you return to your prepregnancy weight sooner. You are also:*

- *less likely to develop high blood pressure and preeclampsia;*
- *have better mental health during your pregnancy, because of the feel-good hormones you produce when active*
- *less likely to have back problems or varicose veins.*

in activity levels as pregnancy continues, means that most women need to increase the amount of calories they consume in only the last trimester, and this is only a modest 300 healthy calories.

However, if you started pregnancy underweight, you may be advised to eat more than usual for the first three months, because this is a critical time for fetal development. If you started pregnancy overweight (BMI 26-30), you should eat healthily and keep active, aiming to keep your weight gain to a minimum until the last trimester.

Later on, if you breastfeed, you will find it energy intensive and recent recommendations are for an extra 335 calories per day for the first six months.

### Expecting twins or more

For twin or multiple pregnancies, it is accepted that there is a need for additional calories and nutrients, and you may need to consume 3,000–3,500 calories per day. Gaining adequate weight in the first 20 weeks predicts a higher birth weight for the babies. See the chart on the facing page for the U.S. Institute of Medicine recommendations on how much to gain for single and twin pregnancies.

## MAKING SAFE FOOD CHOICES

It seems that almost every week there's something new about what we can or can't eat—pregnant or not. While this can be worrying, with a little common sense and some food knowledge, it is simple to avoid what may be risky without denying yourself enjoyable and nutritious foods.

Food safety is important at any stage of life, but while pregnant, extra care is necessary because you and your baby are more vulnerable to illness. By being vigilant about food storage and hygiene, and avoiding just a few foods, you can keep hazards away.

### Cheese

Many cheeses are safe to eat in pregnancy and are a great source of protein, calcium, and phosphorus. The risk from some cheeses is listeriosis, which is a flulike illness that can cause miscarriage or stillbirth.

Cheeses that are safe to eat include:

- All hard cheeses such as American, cheddar, Gouda, Edam, Gruyère, Swiss, etc.
- Hard, unpasteurized varieties, such as Parmesan or Pecorino
- Soft cheeses, such as feta, halloumi, cottage, cream, mascarpone, mozzarella.

However, make sure you avoid:

- Unpasteurized, soft sheep, cow, or goat cheeses

### High protein diets

*It matters in pregnancy where your energy comes from. A healthy pregnancy diet provides a good balance of carbohydrates, fats, and proteins. Eating a high-protein diet means that you will probably have too few carbohydrates and possibly too much fat. The consequences for your baby are still being investigated but there is some evidence that very high intakes of protein could influence a baby's long-term health.*

- Mold-ripened cheese,s such as brie, Camembert, and chevre (a goat cheese);
- Blue-veined cheeses, such as Stilton, gorgonzola, Danish blue, and other blue cheeses, unless you cook them thoroughly, which will kill any listeria bacteria that could be present.

## Fish and shellfish

These highly nutritious foods are good sources of protein, omega 3 fatty acids, and iodine. They should be part of your pregnancy diet but keep in mind:

- All white fish, such as catfish, cod, coley, halibut, pollock, red snapper, sole, and whiting is safe to eat twice a week in 8 ounce portions.
- Oily fish, such as mackerel, salmon, herring, sardines, pilchards, and trout can be eaten up to twice a week in pregnancy.
- Tuna is safe to eat but in limited amounts, because it accumulates some mercury as it ages and grows. Smaller species, such as skipjack or yellowfin, tend to contain less mercury and other pollutants than albacore or "white" tuna. Eat no more than two 6 ounce portions of albacore tuna a week.

### Polychlorinated biphenyls (PCBs)

*You may have heard that some foods, including fish, may contain "persistent organic pollutants" and dioxins. These chemicals are unlikely to pose a major risk to you or your baby, because their level is extremely low and the benefits of eating fish far outweigh the risk of their presence. So don't stop eating fish because of this slim possibility.*

- Some large fish—king mackerel, tilefish, swordfish, and shark—should not be eaten because they can contain methyl mercury.
- Raw fish is not safe to eat because it may contain tiny worms, which are otherwise destroyed when frozen or cooked.
- Check local authorities for advice regarding fish that have been caught in local lakes, rivers, and coastal areas. If they are unsure, one 6 ounce portion per week is the most fish you should eat.

## Nuts and seeds

Peanuts and other nuts, seeds such as sesame, or foods containing them such as peanut butter or tahini, are safe to eat during your pregnancy unless you have an allergy to them or your health professional suggests you avoid them.

## Eggs and foods made with raw eggs

You can eat any style eggs provided the white and yolk are fully cooked. Home-made mayonnaise, sorbets and some desserts such as tiramisu, cold soufflés or mousses made with raw eggs could contain salmonella so are not safe to eat. Shop-bought versions of these are safe to eat. If you are eating out and are unsure whether your meal contains raw egg, make sure to ask.

## Seaweed

If eaten dried or used in breads, seaweed is safe as are red and brown ones often used for sushi. Sushi must be made from frozen fish to be safe to eat. Brown seaweeds, such as kelp and some of the imported Japanese seaweeds, however, are particularly high in iodine, so they should not be eaten.

### BE CAREFUL

*Shellfish, such as mussels, shrimp, and crab, are all fine to eat in pregnancy provided it has been cooked properly so that any bacteria or viruses it may be contaminated with are killed. Raw shellfish, such as oysters or other uncooked shellfish, should not be eaten.*

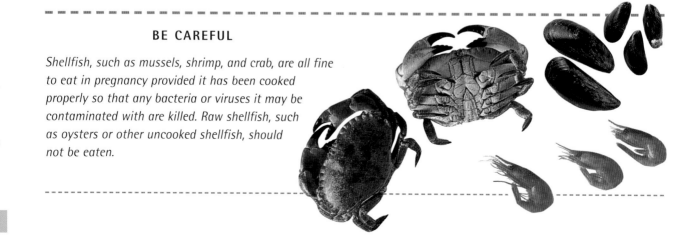

## SAFE FOOD PREPARATION TECHNIQUES

*By following basic food hygiene you can avoid food-borne illnesses that can harm you and your baby.*

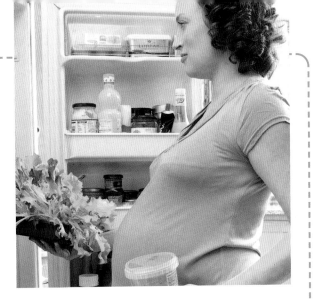

- *Always wash your hands with soap and water before handling food and especially after you have been to the bathroom, handled garbage, touched pets, or changed diapers.*
- *Also wash your hands after handling raw meat, fish, or poultry.*
- *Wear gloves when gardening and if you have a pet, wear gloves to move any animal waste or to change the litter box (better still, have someone else do so). Toxoplasmosis parasites live in animal feces and can cause blindness and brain damage in babies.*
- *Keep your kitchen and food serving area really clean. Bleach cloths and work surfaces regularly; wash dish towels daily and don't use as hand towels.*
- *As soon as possible after shopping, transfer your food to the refrigerator; do not leave it in a warm place, such as the office or car.*
- *Store foods at the right temperature, checking that your refrigerator is below 40°F. The most perishable foods, such as cooked meats, soft cheeses, salad greens, prepared meals, and desserts need to be kept the coolest.*
- *Use the salad crisper at the bottom of your refrigerator for unwashed fruits and vegetables.*
- *Wrap or place in containers any raw meat or fish that may drip onto other foods and place in the coldest part of the refrigerator.*
- *Keep eggs in the refrigerator.*
- *Check expiration and use-by dates on foods and stick to them. Throw out foods that are date expired and don't be tempted to buy reduced short life products at the supermarket.*
- *When preparing foods, keep one board for raw meat and fish and another for cooked foods to prevent cross contamination.*
- *Make sure you wash all fresh fruit before you eat it to reduce the risk of microbial infection, and to remove any dirt or fungicidal sprays. If a fruit has become rotten or moldy, even in one small part, throw it away.*
- *Make sure that when you cook meat it is cooked through. It needs to reach at least 160°F internally, which you can check with a meat thermometer. Another indication is when the juices run clear when you insert a sharp knife to the center of the meat.*

### Liver, liver products, and pâtés

Due to their particularly high levels of vitamin A, which could cause damage to a developing baby, women who are pregnant or planning to become pregnant are advised to avoid all forms of liver and liver products (terrines, pâtés, pastes, etc.) Pâtés that you buy from the delicatessen counter may also be made from other meats, fish, or vegetables, which also are prone to listeria contamination. However, if pâtés have been heat treated by canning, or you make your own being strict with food hygiene, they should be safe.

### Ready-to-eat meals

Foods that have been partly or full prepared for you to reheat at home must be cooked through until piping hot to kill any harmful bacteria.

## Alcohol

Many experts recommend that you do not drink any alcohol during pregnancy. If you choose to drink it, you should have no more than one standard drink at a time no more than once or twice a week. A standard drink is 12 fluid ounces of beer, 5 fluid ounces of wine, and 1½ fluid ounces of 80-proof spirits, such as whiskey, gin, rum, vodka, or tequila. However, the alcohol by volume varies by beverage. To determine the strength of a drink, units are used by UK's Department of Health, which also suggests no alcohol in pregnancy, or limiting alcohol to no more than one or two units once or two times a week. The chart (see right) shows the amounts of units per drink.

If you become pregnant unexpectedly and drank alcohol excessively before you knew you were pregnant, the best advice is to stop drinking and talk to your healthcare provider if you have any concerns.

### The effect of alcohol on your baby

*Alcohol from your bloodstream passes through the placenta to your baby, where his liver breaks it down. However, your baby's liver is not mature enough to do this effectively until you are at least halfway through your pregnancy.*

*It is clear from many studies that heavy drinkers are more likely to have babies who develop fetal alcohol spectrum disorder (FASD) with symptoms such as low birth weight and facial deformities as well as learning difficulties and psychiatric problems.*

*Babies born to binge drinkers (those having more than four drinks of alcohol within two hours) tend to be born prematurely and of low birth weight; there is a higher incidence of miscarriage and stillbirth than for women who don't drink alcohol.*

## Caffeinated beverages

Developing a distaste for coffee can be one of the early signs that you are pregnant, but even if you can still tolerate it, how much should you be drinking while you are expecting or should you give it up altogether? In general, the U.S. Food and Drug Administration (FDA) advises consuming no more than 200 mg of caffeine a day, which is about two

## What is a unit of alcohol?

| Drink and strength (Alcohol by volume ABV) | Amount | Units of alcohol |
|---|---|---|
| White wine 13% | Standard glass 6 fl oz | 2.3 |
| White wine 13% | Large glass 8 fl oz | 3.3 |
| White wine 11% | Standard glass 6 fl oz | 1.9 |
| White wine 11% | Large glass 8 fl oz | 2.8 |
| Champagne 12% | Standard glass 6 fl oz | 2.1 |
| Champagne 12% | Large glass 8 fl oz | 3.0 |
| Red wine 14% | Standard glass 6 fl oz | 2.5 |
| Red wine 14% | Large glass 8 fl oz | 3.5 |
| Red wine 12% | Standard glass 6 fl oz | 2.1 |
| Red wine 12% | Large glass 8 fl oz | 3.0 |
| Rose wine 10% | Standard glass 8 fl oz | 1.8 |
| Rose wine 10% | Large glass 8 fl oz | 2.5 |
| Spirits (gin/vodka) 37.5% | Single shot ¾ fl oz | 0.9 |
| Spirits (gin/vodka) 37.5% | Large single shot 1 fl oz | 1.3 |
| Spirits (gin/vodka) 37.5% | Double shot 1¾ fl oz | 1.9 |
| Alcopop 4% | 700 ml (23⅔ fl oz) bottle | 2.8 |
| Alcopop 4% | 9¼ fl oz bottle | 1.1 |
| Alcopop 5% | 700 ml (23⅔ fl oz) bottle | 3.5 |
| Alcopop 5% | 9¼ fl oz bottle | 1.4 |
| Cider 4.5% | 14¾ fl oz can | 2.0 |
| Cider 7.5% | 9¼ fl oz bottle | 2.1 |
| Cider 7.5% | 17 fl oz can | 3.8 |
| Lager 4% | 11 fl oz bottle | 1.3 |
| Lager 4% | 14¾ fl oz can | 1.8 |
| Lager 5% | 14¾ fl oz can | 2.2 |

5 fluid ounce cups of coffee. The American College of Obstetricians and Gynecologists advises women that are planning a pregnancy or are pregnant to keep their caffeine intake to no more than 200 mg, or two small 5 fluid ounce cups of coffee a day. Studies have shown that large intakes of caffeine can be linked to infertility, low birth weight babies, and miscarriage.

When considering your caffeine intake, it's important to keep in mind that caffeine is not only found in coffee, tea, and cola, but also in energy drinks, chocolate, and cocoa as well as in many cold and flu remedies.

With chocolate, the darker the chocolate, the higher the amount of caffeine, although in real terms this is not significant unless you are eating several bars of chocolate each day. As you may know from the coffee shops you visit, the strength of the brew may be determined by the barista. In Great Britain, the Food Standards Agency Food Surveillance Unit has measured caffeine levels in beverages, both brewed domestically as well as in the laboratory. Not surprisingly, there are differences and these are shown by the range of measurements in the chart (see left).

Manufacturers of energy drinks that contain more than 150 mg of caffeine per liter, must declare their caffeine content in Europe, but because caffeine is not a nutrient, it does not need to be stated on food or drink labels in the United States. As you can see from the chart, an energy drink may contain less caffeine than a cup of coffee, but it will add to your caffeine intake. It is important that you are aware of the amount of caffeine in a range of products so you know how much you are consuming throughout the day.

Decaffeinated coffees and teas are great alternatives in pregnancy and you may also want to try herb or fruit teas. They can be refreshing and some have benefits of their own. Chamomile is said to enhance sleep and peppermint aids digestion. Raspberry leaf tea is reputed to ease labor and strengthen the uterus when taken in the last trimester, but don't drink it before then, because it has been linked to miscarriage.

My book, *Superdrinks for Pregnancy*, provides a lot of delicious and healthy alternatives to caffeinated and alcoholic drinks.

## Comparison of caffeine-containing items

| Item | Quantity (approx.) | Estimated amount of caffeine/Source |
|---|---|---|
| Instant coffee | One mug (8¾ fl oz) | 100* |
| | One cup (6½ fl oz) | 75* |
| Black tea, infusion | One mug (8¾ fl oz) | 50-75* |
| | One cup (6½ fl oz) | 33-50* |
| hot cocoa mix | Made as per package directions (6¾ fl oz) | 1.1-8.2* |
| Filter coffee | Small (7⅔ fl oz) | 160+ |
| | Medium (12 fl oz) | 240+ |
| | Large (15 fl oz) | 320+ |
| Cappuccino or latte | Small (7⅔ fl oz) | 75+ |
| | Medium (12 fl ml) | 75+ |
| | Large (15 fl oz) | 150+ |
| Mocha | Small (7⅔ fl oz) | 90+ |
| | Medium (12 fl oz) | 95+ |
| | Large (15 fl oz) | 175+ |
| Flat white | Small (7⅔ fl oz) | 150 |
| Americano coffee | Small (7⅔ fl oz) | 75+ |
| | Medium (12 fl oz) | 150+ |
| | Large (15 fl oz) | 225+ |
| Energy drink (Red Bull) | 16 fl oz can | 151^ |
| Cola beverages | 11 fl oz can | 11-70* |
| 70 percent dark chocolate | 1⅜ oz | 6@ |
| Milk chocolate | 1⅜ oz | 3@ |
| Unsweetened cocoa powder | As made 6½ fl oz cup | <1@ |

* FSA Survey of Caffeine Levels in Hot Beverages, Food Information Sheet 53/04 April 2004, and FSA 2008
+ Starbucks nutritional information accessed March 2011. @ Green and Black's Organic Chocolate accessed March 2011 ^ Calculated from label

## FOOD AND COMMON PREGNANCY DISCOMFORTS

Some lucky women will sail through pregnancy with no complications and really are the picture of health. For others, however, pregnancy involves a range of health issues. Some can be managed by making changes to what and how you eat. Many of the more minor conditions are thought to be caused by the huge hormonal upheaval that characterizes early pregnancy. Indeed, an aversion to certain foods can be one of the first signs of pregnancy.

### Cravings and aversions

It is estimated that more than half of all pregnant women are affected by these, and the reasons why are not fully understood. One theory, which makes logical sense, is that if you experience nausea and vomiting while eating or drinking, it could be because your body is protecting your baby from potential harmful toxins. Aversions to coffee, meat, eggs, spicy foods, and some vegetables are not uncommon, and generally shouldn't put you at a nutritional disadvantage if you find alternative nutrient-rich foods. So, for example, if you can't eat meat, try fish or other zinc- and iron-rich foods. If you can't drink coffee, try herbal tisanes instead.

Cravings, on the other hand, were once thought to be a sign that your body had a nutritional need. While this might be the true for commonly craved foods such as broccoli, milk, or grapefruit, it does not explain some women's craving for nonfoods, such as coal, ice, or soil. Neither is there a nutritional need in craving low-nutrient foods, such as chocolate, cakes, and cookies. If you do want these kinds of foods, but are otherwise following a healthy diet, then go ahead and have a small portion. Just make sure that they don't fill you and replace more nutritious foods.

### Sickness and nausea

Both are early indicators of pregnancy and are not necessarily limited to the morning. The peak of sickness and nausea is usually around 6 to 18 weeks when your baby is particularly vulnerable, so they may be your body's ways of preventing you consuming foods, which could cause damage or promote miscarriage. A comprehensive review of various methods used to alleviate nausea done in

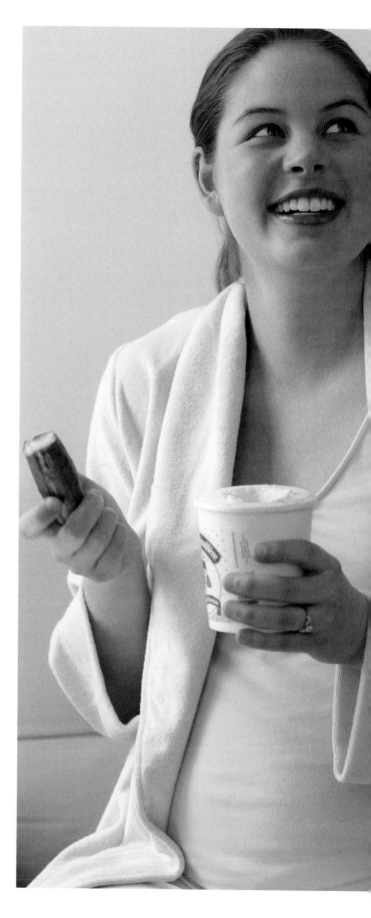

2010 found that using ginger or vitamin $B_6$ were most effective.

- Have a slice of ginger root in hot water as your first drink of the day.
- Use fresh or ground ginger in your cooking.
- Sip on ginger ale if you can tolerate the bubbles.
- Have a ginger supplement—up to 1 g is safe.
- Have a vitamin $B_6$ supplement—up to 50 mg is safe.

## Heartburn

You may find that as you pregnancy progresses you experience a burning sensation in your throat, because acid from your stomach is forced up the esophagus. As with many pregnancy problems, it is caused by changes in your hormones, which relax the muscles controlling the valve at the entry to your stomach. As your baby grows, he will also "squash" your internal organs. However, there are some things to try:

- Avoid or limit chocolate, spicy or fatty foods, coffee, tea, and carbonated or acidic beverages (such as fruit juice).
- Drink low-fat milk to help "settle" your stomach.
- Eat frequent small meals instead of a few large ones, and sit down for a while afterward.
- Sleep more upright; prop yourself up with pillows.

## Constipation

With this common pregnancy problem, prevention is far preferable to "cure," so make sure that you drink plenty of water and eat fiber-rich whole grain cereals and vegetables.

- Carry (and drink from) a water bottle so you don't become dehydrated.
- Add lentils and beans to soups, stews, and curries.

- Stick a package of apricots, figs, or prunes into your bag to nibble on.
- Use whole-wheat bread, whole-grain cereals, and opt for high-fiber muesli.
- Have baked beans on whole-wheat toast or a baked potato with skin for a quick high-fiber lunch.
- Have peas and/or corn as regular vegetables.

## Pregnancy diabetes

Also known as gestational diabetes, it is caused by your body failing to produce enough of the hormone insulin to control your blood glucose (sugar). Your need for insulin increases in pregnancy, and if you are not making enough, you will have too much glucose in your bloodstream and it will pass through the placenta to your baby. This is dangerous for you and your baby and increases the risk that your baby will be large for her gestational age. You could also have other complications in pregnancy and labor unless the diabetes is properly managed. Adopting a healthy lifestyle throughout pregnancy will not only reduce your risk of developing the condition, but will also help you to manage it if you do develop it.

- Be particularly careful to eat whole-grain and minimally processed cereals, concentrating on low GI foods (see page 20).
- Avoid drinks that are high in sugars, whether natural or not, especially between meals.
- Plan your meals to include a source of protein, some vegetables, and a low to medium GI carbohydrate food, such as plain boiled potatoes, pearl barley, or basmati rice.
- Avoid snacking on cakes, cookies, ice cream, or confectionery.

### CHAPTER 4

# MENU PLANS

A great deal of thought and hard work has gone into the creation of the recipes. My brief was to create healthy dishes—full of the nutrients that pregnant and new moms need—but also that taste great. But even with this array of dishes, it can be complicated to create varied meal plans that meet all your daily requirements. So to ensure you and your baby benefit from the right nutrients at the right times, I've devised special meal plans.

There are four different plans—one for each trimester and one for the newborn weeks. Each plan contains breakfasts, lunches, dinners, snacks, and drinks to make sure that your diet is varied, interesting, and meets your specific requirements for the stage. Recipes from the book are italicized, while the other suggestions can be store bought; all the selections ensure that your diet remains varied and interesting.

## FIRST TRIMESTER

During the first few weeks of pregnancy, a lot is going on as your body adapts to your new state and your baby develops. All this development—your baby grows from a few microscopic cells to a being with all his or her major organs and systems—and the hormonal changes required to nourish the placenta, can make you feeling exhausted, especially if you are especially nauseous or sick. By following my menu plan, you will keep well-nourished, but if you can't stomach regular meals, the "Little plates" provides a range of small nutritious meals and snacks.

Tiredness can also be due to anemia, a lack of iron, or occasionally vitamin $B_{12}$ or folic acid. If you didn't have a particularly good diet before pregnancy, are vegan, or don't eat much meat, especially red meat, then it may be worth having your iron stores checked. A simple blood test reveals it.

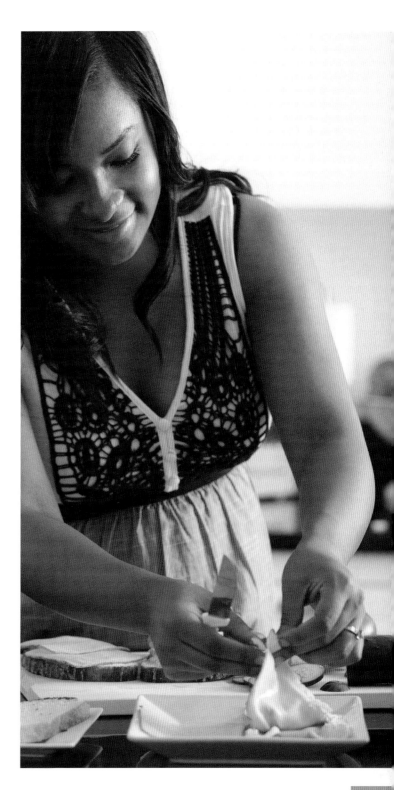

If you are vomiting, it is important to replace the lost fluids by drinking plenty. It doesn't matter if it is water, herbal tea, milk, or diluted fruit juice. If you consume caffeine, regular tea or coffee is fine but in limited amounts (see page 34). Some women find ginger helpful in alleviating nausea and it may work for you. Ask your partner to bring you a cup of hot water with a slice of fresh ginger root to bed in the morning, accompanied perhaps by a gingernut or plain cookie. Recipes that use ginger include: Teriyaki Turkey with Sesame Cucumber Salad (page 95) and Sea Bass with Pomegranate Salsa (page 114).

## SECOND TRIMESTER

By now you may be starting to feel a little more energetic and may have regained your appetite, because the nausea will probably have diminished. Although your calorie needs haven't yet increased, its important you follow my menu plan in order to eat the nutrient-rich foods that make sure your baby has enough vitamins and minerals for her development. Having extra energy, means its a good idea to cook some meals in bulk and freeze them. When your baby arrives, you will be both busy and tired and cooking will probably not be a priority, so whether you or your partner do the cooking, get ahead with a little planning. You'll appreciate the few extra minutes that you spend chopping and cooking now when you are time-poor in the weeks after the birth.

If you haven't started to take vitamin D supplements, now is the time to do so, especially if you don't get out in the sun much, have dark skin, or cover your skin for cultural reasons.

Try to eat more vitamin D-rich foods. Althoung not many foods actually provide it, several of my recipes—Smoked Salmon Flakes with Herbed Lentils (page 116), Tuna Steaks with Sun-Dried Tomato Crust and Lime Dressing (page 119), Mushroom and Asparagus Omelet (page 55), Grilled Sardine and Cheese Sandwich (page 69), and Herrings with Avocado and Cherry Tomatoes (page 117)—provide at least one-quarter of your day's needs.

Another great way of getting vitamin D is to enjoy a little sunshine—half an hour a day before 11 a.m. or after 3 p.m. will top up your stores without increasing your risk of cancer.

## THIRD TRIMESTER

Your baby's brain and nervous system need the whole of your pregnancy to grow and mature, but in this trimester the process of myelination occurs, when a fatty sheath insulates nervous system. This requires the presence of vitamin $B_{12}$ as well as an adequate supply (200 mg day) of the omega 3 fatty acid, DHA (docosahexaenoic acid). Making sure you have some oily fish at least once but not more than twice a week will provide your baby with DHA . My menu plan and a variety of recipes in the book (see page 154) will ensure that it is the case.

If you don't eat fish, eat omega 3-fortified eggs or milk, sprinkle flaxseed on cereals or salads, or as use a flaxseed pressed oil in salad dressings. Omega 6 fatty acids, unfortunatel,y compete with omega 3s for absorption in the body, so if you don't eat fish and rely on vegetarian sources for your omega 3, it's best not to have too much omega 6 in your diet. Because sunflower spreads and oil are the most common source of omega 6 in the diet, simply use monounsaturate-

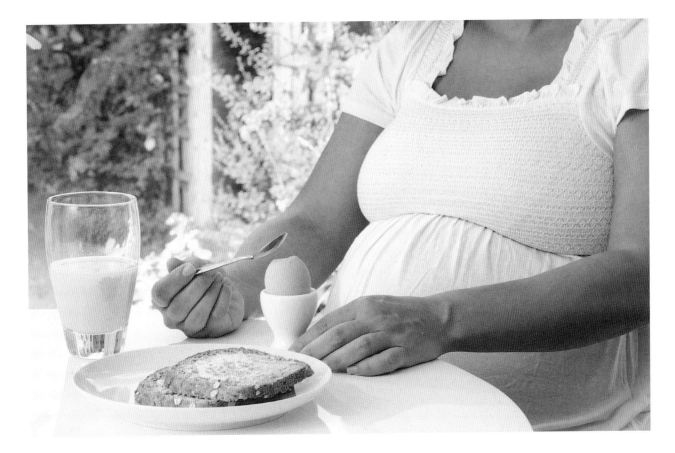

rich oils and spreads, such as canola and olive instead of polyunsaturated sunflower, corn, or peanut oils.

As your baby grows bigger, she will start to squash some of your internal organs and the digestive tract, and this can cause you to become constipated. To avoid this, drink plenty of fluids, at least six to eight cups of water or other fluids each day, keep active, and top up on fiber-rich foods, such as Raspberry Oatmeal with Walnuts (page 51), Orange Bran Muffins (page 151), Fruity Oat Bars (page 149), and Herbed Barley (page 138). Eating normal size portions may again be difficult, so look at my "Little Plates" recipes, which will give you the essential nutrients without filling you up too much.

## BREASTFEEDING AND THE EARLY WEEKS WITH YOUR NEW BABY

Whether or not you are breastfeeding, you need to eat nourishing foods and rest when you can. If you are breastfeeding, you must make sure that your increased need for vitamins and minerals is met. My menu plan makes sures this is the case.

Perhaps not surprisingly one of the greatest increases is in the amount of calcium you need. Try to have calcium-rich snacks and milky drinks, such as malted milk, cocoa, or plain hot milk, when you sit down to feed your baby. Also prepare my recipes that use tofu, cheese, milk, or yogurt, or contain canned fish with bones, such as Berry Yogurt Breakfast (page 53), Bean and Salsa Wrap (page 68), Baba Ganoush (page 56), Roasted Baby Vegetables with Tofu (page 124), Crab Cakes with Watercress and Orange Salad (page 111), and Baked Figs with Pistachio and Honeyed Yogurt (page 146), because these all supply calcium, and many provide magnesium, zinc, copper, and the B vitamins, all needed in greater quantities.

Some babies who develop colic do seem to improve when their mother avoids certain foods. The culprits usually cited are garlic, onions, foods from the cabbage family, citrus fruits, and even chocolate. So if you suspect your baby is unsettled when you eat one of these foods, omit it for a couple of days and see if there is an improvement. Talk to your healthcare provider if you are intending to make this kind of change to make sure you don't accidentally leave crucial nutrient-rich foods out of your diet.

# FIRST TRIMESTER

| | | Monday | Tuesday | Wednesday |
|---|---|---|---|---|
| **breakfast** | | • Raspberry Oatmeal with Walnuts OR<br>• Bran Flakes with golden raisins OR<br>• Scrambled egg on whole-wheat toast with broiled tomatoes<br>PLUS<br>• Orange juice | • 2 boiled eggs with whole-wheat roll and spread OR<br>• Muesli with extra fruit OR<br>• Greek yogurt with strawberries and honey<br>PLUS<br>• Berry smoothie (page 40) | • Muesli with yogurt and raspberries OR<br>• 2 Weetabix with blueberries OR<br>• Greek yogurt, fruit, and seeds<br>PLUS<br>• Orange juice |
| **lunch** | | • Greens soup OR<br>• Carrot and cilantro soup WITH<br>• Watercress and Salmon Salad OR<br>• Egg, Tomato, and Onion Roll<br><br>• Low fat fruit yogurt | • Romaine, Chicken, and Crouton Salad OR<br>• Ratatouille with Cheese and Bread OR<br>• Baked beans on 2 slices whole-wheat toast with spread<br><br>• 2 clementines OR<br>• 1 slice fresh pineapple | • Smoked Mackerel, Ricotta, and Beet Bruschetta OR<br>• Pasta Primavera OR<br>• Beef and Beet Sandwich<br><br>• Carrot Sheet Cake OR<br>• Chocolate Brazil Brownie |
| **dinner** | | • Sesame and Cilantro Chicken with Mango Salsa OR<br>• Greek-Style Tomato and Haddock OR<br>• Black-Eyed Pea, Dried Currant, and Fresh Mint Stew WITH<br>• Almond Rice OR<br>• Hot Potato Salad AND<br>• Steamed snowpeas OR<br>• Watercress and baby greens salad with fat-free French dressing<br><br>• Baked Fig with Pistachios and Honey Yogurt OR<br>• Strawberry Mousse | • Creamy Vegetarian Ground "Beef" WITH Herbed Barley OR<br>• Hungarian Goulash WITH Leek Potatoes OR<br>• Chocolate and Chile Chicken WITH Quinoa and Sunflower Seeds WITH<br>• Green Chile Edamame OR<br>• Steamed broccoli<br><br>• Mango and Lime Dessert OR<br>• Summer Fruit Compote (with xylitol) with 1 scoop vanilla ice cream | • Turkey Herb Burger with Fruity Salsa OR<br>• Vegetable Crepes with Red Pepper Sauce OR<br>• Sausage and Orzo Stew WITH<br>• Steamed broccoli<br><br>• 2 plums OR<br>• 1 pear |
| **snacks** | | • ¼ cup dried apricots<br>• Carrot Sheet Cake | • Fruity Oat Bar<br>• 1 plain cookie OR<br>• 6 chocolate-covered Brazil nuts | • Apple OR orange |

**DRINKS:** 1¼ cups low-fat milk or fortified soy equivalent in drinks throughout the day. Water ad lib throughout the day, and herb tea, coffee, and tea as guided by chapter 3. Fruit juice assumed to be 7 to 8 fl oz glass unsweetened.

| Thursday | Friday | Saturday | Sunday |
|---|---|---|---|
| • *Mushroom and Asparagus Omelet* OR<br>• *Raisin and Apple Pancakes* OR<br>• Dried fruit roll and banana PLUS<br>• *Orange and Pomegranate Salad* | • 2 boiled eggs with whole-wheat roll and spread OR<br>• Homemade oatmeal OR<br>• 2 Weetabix with raisins WITH<br>• Whole-grain toast and spread PLUS<br>• Strawberry smoothie | • *Mexican Brunch* OR<br>• *Dried Fruit Salad* OR<br>• Croissant or crescent roll with preserves and clementine PLUS<br>• Skinny cappuccino | • Muesli with yogurt and raspberries OR<br>• Bran flakes with dried apricots OR<br>• Dried fruit roll with spread and banana PLUS<br>• Mango and peach smoothie |
| • *Barley and Roasted Vegetable Salad with Pumpkins Seeds* OR<br>• *Bean and Salsa Wrap* OR<br>• Scrambled egg on toast with broiled tomatoes | • *Moroccan Hummus with Flatbread* OR<br>• *Quinoa, Feta, and Spinach Salad* OR<br>• Cheddar and tomato sandwich in sunflower seed roll<br><br>• *Citrus Salad Bowl* | • Store-bought "healthier" vegetable pizza OR<br>• Smoked salmon and cream cheese bagel OR<br>• *Grilled Sardine and Cheese Sandwich*<br><br>• Greek yogurt with strawberries and honey OR<br>• Fresh mango | • *Homemade Fish Sticks with Piquant Avocado Dip* OR<br>• *Baba Ganoush with Bread and Asparagus Tips* WITH<br>• *Sardine and Pepper Strudels* OR<br>• *Tzatziki with Raw Vegetables* AND<br>• *Two Pear Salad* OR<br>• *Patatas Bravas*<br><br>• Papaya with lime juice OR<br>• *Summer Fruit Compote* (with xylitol) |
| • *Tuna Steak with Sun-Dried Tomato Crust and Lime Dressing* OR<br>• *Pot Roasted Lamb Shanks* OR<br>• *Stuffed Portobello Mushrooms* WITH<br>• *Gratin of Potato* OR<br>• Plain cooked pasta AND<br>• *Spinach with Dried Currants and Pine Nuts* OR<br>• Green salad with dressing<br><br>• Slice of cantaloupe or honeydew melon OR<br>• 2 Kiwifruit | • Watercress soup<br>• Steak and Broccoli with Noodles OR<br>• Asparagus risotto OR<br>• Italian Chicken Gnocchi<br><br>• *Chocolate Brioche Pudding* OR<br>• *Honey-Roasted Stone Fruit* | • *Tarka Dhal* WITH<br>• *Almond Rice* OR<br>• *Salmon and Asparagus en Croûte* WITH<br>• *Hot Potato Salad* OR<br>• *Teriyaki Turkey* WITH<br>• *Quinoa and Sunflower Seeds* AND<br>• *Curly Kale with Garlic Cherry Tomatoes* OR<br>• Peas and carrots<br><br>• *Strawberry Mousse* OR<br>• *Citrus Salad Bowl* | • *Crab Linguine* OR<br>• *Baked Beef and Sour Cherries* WITH brown rice OR<br>• *Baked Butternut Squash with Cheese and Pomegranate* WITH<br>• Watercress and orange salad OR<br>• Peas and carrots OR<br>• Green salad with dressing<br><br>• *Apple and Black Currant Oat Crisp* OR<br>• *Traditional Rice Pudding* |
| • Glass of milk<br>• *Orange Bran Muffin* | • Mango OR papaya<br>• *Fruity Oat Bar* | • 6 chocolate Brazil nuts | • ½ cup dried fruit, nuts, and seeds<br>• Fruit yogurt |

**NOTES:** Portion of vegetables or fruit is about 3 oz or more unless specified. Where lower fat options exist, assume these are used. All spread assumed to be reduced fat (60%) olive spread. Yogurt is low fat unless stated. Mayonnaise is 3% fat and only 1 tablespoon is used in sandwiches. Bread is an average slice of 1 oz, 2 slices per sandwich. Salad dressing is assumed to be 1 tablespoon standard French dressing.

# SECOND TRIMESTER

| | Monday | Tuesday | Wednesday |
|---|---|---|---|
| **breakfast** | • *Oatmeals with Raspberries and Walnuts* OR<br>• *Citrus Salad Bowl* OR<br>• Bran flakes with apricots<br><br>• Pineapple-based smoothie | • Scrambled egg with tomatoes and toast OR<br>• Muesli with blueberries OR<br>• *Berry Yogurt Greakfast*<br><br>• Apple OR orange juice | • *Berry Yogurt Breakfast* OR<br>• Boiled eggs with marmite on toast OR<br>• *Orange Bran Muffin* WITH<br>• Glass of milk AND<br>• *Citrus Salad Bowl* |
| **lunch** | • Peanut butter and watercress sandwich OR<br>• *Beef and Beet Sandwich* OR<br>• *Quinoa, Feta, and Spinach Salad*<br><br>• 1 orange OR some mango cubes | • Baked beans on 2 pieces toast OR<br>• Greens soup with cheese roll OR<br>• *Smoked Mackerel, Ricotta, and Beet Bruschetta*<br><br>• Half papaya with lime juice OR<br>• Large kiwifruit | • *Grilled Sardine and Cheese Sandwich* OR<br>• Baked potato with tuna OR<br>• *Bean and Salsa Wrap* WITH<br>• Green salad and dressing<br><br>• Grapes OR prunes |
| **dinner** | • *Crab Linguine* OR<br>• *Aparagus Risotto* OR<br>• *Jambalaya* WITH<br>• Green salad with dressing OR<br>• Green beans and chorizo<br><br>• *Chocolate Brazil Brownie* OR<br>• *Honey-Roasted Stone Fruit* | • *Tuna Steak with Sun-Dried Tomato Crust and Lime Dressing* OR<br>• *Duck with Cherries and Leek Mashed Potatoes* OR<br>• *Brazil Nut Burger* in bun WITH<br>• *Kachumbari* OR<br>• *Roast Beet and Butternut Squash* AND<br>• *Orange and Mint Couscous* OR<br>• *Hot Potato Salad*<br><br>• *Strawberry Mousse* OR<br>• *Mango and Lime Dessert* | • *Baked Butternut Squash with Cheese and Pomegranate* OR<br>• *Roasted Pork Balls and Vegetables* OR<br>• *Duck with Cherries and Leek Mashed Potatoes* WITH<br>• *Green Chile Edamame* OR<br>• *Curly Kale with Garlic Cherry Tomatoes*<br><br>• *Pear in Chocolate Sauce* OR<br>• *Raspberry and Pomegranate Jelly* |
| **snacks** | • Fruit yogurt<br>• *Fruity Oat Bar* | • *Carrot Sheet Cake* | • *Cheddar and Sun-Dried Tomato Biscuit* |

**DRINKS:** 1¼ cups low-fat or fortified soy equivalent in drinks throughout the day. Water ad lib throughout the day, and herb tea, coffee, and tea as guided by chapter 3. Fruit juice assumed to be 7 to 8 fl oz glass unsweetened.

| Thursday | Friday | Saturday | Sunday |
|---|---|---|---|
| • Mango, apricot, and pineapple smoothie with dreid fruit bread OR<br>• *Orange Bran Muffin* WITH<br>• Glass of milk OR<br>• *Raspberry Oatmeals with Walnuts* | • *Raisin and Apple Pancakes* OR<br>• Weetabix with raisins OR<br>• Muesli with blueberries AND<br>• Berry smoothie | • Croissant or crescent roll and preserves with clementines OR<br>• *Orange Bran Muffin* WITH<br>• Glass of milk OR<br>• *Raspberry Oatmeal with Walnuts* | • *Mexican Brunch* OR<br>• Weetabix with raisins OR<br>• *Raspberry Oatmeal with Walnuts* AND<br>• Orange juice |
| • *Barley and Roasted Vegetable Salad with Pumpkins Seeds* OR<br>• *Beef and Beet Sandwich* OR<br>• Carrot and cilantro soup and whole-wheat roll<br><br>• Apple juice | • *Crab Cakes with Watercress and Orange Salad* OR<br>• *Mushroom and Asparagus Omelee* OR<br>• *Ratatouille with Cheese and Bread* WITH<br>• *Chile Edamame and Peppers* OR<br>• *Cucumber and Sesame Salad* | • *Stuffed Portobello Mushrooms* OR<br>• *Watercress and salmon salad* OR<br>• *Baba Ganoush with Bread and Asparagus Tips* WITH<br>• Green salad and dressing<br><br>• Slice of melon or an apple | • Greens soup with cheese roll OR<br>• Boiled eggs with whole-wheat roll OR<br>• *Grilled Sardine and Cheese Sandwich* WITH<br>• Cherry tomatoes<br><br>• *Fruity Oat Bar* OR<br>• *Carrot Sheet Cake* |
| • *Herrings with Avocado and Tomato Salad* OR<br>• *Beef in Beer* OR<br>• *Spinach Stuffed Chicken Breast with Proscuitto* WITH<br>• *Herbed Barley* OR<br>• *Leek Potatoes* AND<br>• *Spinach with Dried Currants and Peanuts*<br><br>• *Summer Fruit Compote* OR<br>• Plums | • *Water Chestnut and Cashew Nut Stir Fry* OR<br>• *Chorizo and Black-Eyed Peas with Israeli Couscous* OR<br>• *Paella* WITH<br>• Sweet AND<br>• Broccoli with Almonds and Sun-Dried Tomatoes<br><br>• *Pear in Chocolate Sauce* OR<br>• *Chocolate Brazil Brownie* | • *Black-Eyed Peas, Dried Currant, and Fresh Mint Stew* OR<br>• *Sea Bass with Pomegranate Salsa* OR<br>• *Hungarian Goulash* WITH<br>• New potatoes OR<br>• Brown rice AND<br>• *Roasted Beet and Butternut Squash* OR<br>• Broccoli with Amonds<br><br>• *Orange and Pomegranate Salad* OR<br>• Greek yogurt, blueberries, and honey | • *Pot Roasted Lamb Shanks* OR<br>• *Roasted Baby Vegetables with Tofu* OR<br>• *Tuna Steak with Sun-Dried Tomato Crust and Lime Dressing* WITH<br>• *Hot Potato Salad* OR<br>• *Gratin of Potato* AND<br>• Baby broccoli<br><br>• Tropical fruit salad OR<br>• Yogurt with blueberries<br>• Raspberries |
| • Plain cookie | • Grapes OR Kiwifruit<br>• Chocolate Brazils | • Mango and passion fruit smoothie | • Prunes<br>• *Cheddar and Sun-Dried Tomato Biscuits* |

NOTES: Portion of vegetables or fruit is about 3 oz or more unless specified. Where lower fat options exist, assume these are used. All spread assumed to be reduced fat (60%) olive spread. Yogurt is low fat unless stated. Mayonnaise is 3% fat and only 1 tablespoon is used in sandwiches. Bread is an average slice of 1 oz, 2 slices per sandwich. Salad dressing is assumed to be 1 tablespoon standard French dressing.

# THIRD TRIMESTER

| | | Monday | Tuesday | Wednesday |
|---|---|---|---|---|
| **breakfast** | | • 2 boiled eggs with whole-wheat toast OR<br>• Bran flakes with dried apricots OR<br>• 2 wheat biscuits with blueberries<br><br>• Glass of orange juice | • Muesli with blueberries OR<br>• 2 wheat biscuits with raisins OR<br>• 2 boiled eggs with marmite on toast<br><br>• Glass of orange juice | • Smoked salmon and cream cheese bagel OR<br>• *Raspberry Oatmeal with Walnuts* OR<br>• Cheerios<br><br>• Glass of orange juice |
| **lunch** | | • Scrambled egg with broiled tomatoes and toast OR<br>• Baked potato with tuna OR<br>• Cheddar and tomato sunflower seed roll<br><br>• 2 clemetines AND<br>• 1 fruit yogurt | • *Homemade Fish Sticks with Piquant Avocado Dip* OR<br>• *Roasted Red Pepper Paté* with multigrain bread OR<br>• Smoked mackerel paté and cucumber sandwich<br><br>• *Carrot Sheet Cake* | • Peanut butter and watercress sandwich OR<br>• Shrimp and cucumber sandwich OR<br>• Mushroom soup with a few chopped walnuts and a whole-wheat roll<br><br>• Greek yogurt with strawberries and honey AND<br>• 1 plain cookie |
| **dinner** | | • *Mushroom-Stuffed Chicken with Green Lentils* OR<br>• *Crab Cakes with Watercress and Orange Salad* OR<br>• *Brazil Nut Burger* in a roll WITH<br>• *Ginger and Orange Slaw* OR<br>• *Roasted Beet and Butternut Squash* AND<br>• *Orange and Mint Couscous*<br><br>• 2 scoops ice cream OR<br>• 1 scoop with *Summer Fruit Compote* | • *Greek-Style Tomato and Fish* OR<br>• *Pork with Pineapple* OR<br>• *Black-Eyed Pea, Dried Currant, and Fresh Mint Stew* WITH<br>• *Leek Potatoes* OR<br>• *Almond Rice* AND<br>• *Watercress and Orange Salad* OR<br>• *Broccoli with Almonds*<br><br>• *Traditional Rice Pudding* OR<br>• *Baked Fig with Pistachios and Honey Yogurt* | • *Pasta Primavera* OR<br>• *Tuna and Vegetable Pasta Casserole* OR<br>• *Italian Chicken Gnocchi* WITH<br>• Broccoli or carrots<br><br>• *Strawberry Mousse* |
| **snacks** | | • 1 oz bag low fat potato chips<br>• *Cheddar and Sun-Dried Tomato Biscuit*<br>• *Fruity Oat Bar* | • Glass of milk<br>• *Chocolate Brazil Brownie* | • Glass of milk<br>• *Fruity Oat Bar* |

**DRINKS:** 1¼ cups low-fat milk or fortified soy equivalent in drinks throughout the day. Water ad lib throughout the day, and herb tea, coffee, and tea as guided by chapter 3. Fruit juice assumed to be 7 to 8 fl oz glass unsweetened.

| Thursday | Friday | Saturday | Sunday |
|---|---|---|---|
| • Shredded wheat with strawberries OR<br>• *Orange Bran Muffin* WITH<br>• Glass of milk OR<br>• Croissant or crescent roll and preserves WITH<br>• Clementine | • Greek yogurt, blueberries, and honey OR<br>• Croissant or crescent roll and preserves WITH<br>• Clementine OR<br>• Bran flakes with raisins<br><br>• Berry smoothie OR<br>• Chai masala | • Broiled bacon, tomatoes, and mushrooms OR<br>• *Orange Bran Muffin* AND<br>• Glass of milk OR<br>• *Raspberry Oatmeal with Walnuts* AND<br>• Slice of toast and spread<br><br>• Glass of orange juice | • *Mexican Brunch* OR<br>• Shredded wheat with strawberries OR<br>• Croissant or crescent roll and preserves WITH<br>• Clementine<br>• ½ grapefruit |
| • *Morrocan Hummus with Flatbread* OR<br>• Homemade vegetable pizza OR<br>• Ham salad sandwich with seeded bread<br><br>• 2 kiwifruit or 3 plums | • *Sardine and Pepper Strudel* OR<br>• 2 boiled eggs with marmite on toast OR<br>• Turkey and cranberry salad sandwich<br>AND<br>• Yogurt with berries OR<br>• Papaya with lime<br><br>• *Chocolate Brazil Brownie* | • *Smoked Mackerel, Ricotta, and Beet Bruschetta* OR<br>• *Romaine, Chicken, and Croutons Salad* OR<br>• 2 boiled eggs with marmite on toast<br><br>• Mango cubes OR<br>• 3 dried apricots | • Carrot and cilantro soup with a roll OR<br>• Smoked salmon and cream cheese bagel OR<br>• *Moroccan Houmous with Flatbread* WITH<br>• Green salad |
| • *Stuffed Portobello Mushrooms* OR<br>• *Baked Beef and Sour Cherries* OR<br>• *Greek-Style Tomato and Fish* WITH<br>• *Hot Potato Salad* OR<br>• *Tabbouleh with Pine Nuts* AND<br>• *Two Pear Salad*<br><br>• *Pear in Chocolate Sauce* OR<br>• *Raisin and Apple Pancake* | • *Smoked Salmon Flakes with Herbed Lentils* OR<br>• *Duck and Asian Mushroom Stir-Fry* OR<br>• *Water Chestnut and Cashew Stir-Fry*<br><br>• *Strawberry Mousse* OR<br>• *Mango and Lime Dessert* | • *Beef in Beer* OR<br>• *Lamb and Pepper Skewers with Tzatziki* OR<br>• *Mushroom and Asparagus Omelet* WITH<br>• *Gratin Potatoes* OR<br>• Pasta AND<br>• *Broccoli with Almonds* OR<br>• *Spinach with Dried Currants and Pine Nuts* | • Duck with *Cherries and Leek Mashed Potatoes* OR<br>• *Moroccan Lamb Stew* OR<br>• *Roasted Baby Vegetables with Tofu* WITH<br>• *Orange and Mint Couscous* AND<br>• Peas AND<br>• *Curly Kale with Garlic Cherry Tomatoes*<br><br>• *Traditional Rice Pudding* OR<br>• *2 scoops ice cream* |
| • *Cheddar and Sun-Dried Tomato Biscuit*<br>• Glass of orange juice | • Cappuccino<br>• *Moroccan Hummus with Flatbread* | • Greek yogurt and blueberries<br>• Hot spicy apple drink | • Glass of milk<br>• Pineapple, banana, and ginger smoothie |

**NOTES:** Portion of vegetables or fruit is 3 oz or more unless specified. Where lower fat options exist, assume these are used. All spread assumed to be reduced fat (60%) olive spread. Yogurt is low fat unless stated. Mayonnaise is 3% fat and only 1 tablespoon is used in sandwiches. Bread is an average slice of 1 oz, 2 slices per sandwich. Salad dressing is assumed to be 1 tablespoon standard French dressing.

# NEWBORN WEEKS

| | | Monday | Tuesday | Wednesday |
|---|---|---|---|---|
| **breakfast** | | • Oat and wheat flakes with dried fruit OR<br>• *Raspberry Oatmeal with Walnuts* OR<br>• *Mexican Brunch* | • *Orange bran muffin* OR<br>• Weetabix with blueberries OR<br>• Boiled eggs with whole-wheat roll<br><br>• Orange juice | • *Raisin and apple pancakes* OR<br>• *Raspberry Oatmeal with Walnuts* OR<br>• Muesli with blueberries<br><br>• Orange juice |
| **lunch** | | • Baked potato with tuna mixed with mayonnaise OR<br>• *Grilled Sardine and Cheese Sandwich* OR<br>• *Beef and Beet Sandwich*<br><br>• Banana or dried apricots | • *Carrot soup with roll* OR<br>• *Tuna and Vegetabe Pasta Casserole* OR<br>• Scrambled eggs with broiled tomato and toast<br><br>• Apple | • *Smoked Salmon Flakes with Herbed Lentils* OR<br>• *Grilled Sardine and Cheese Sandwich* OR<br>• *Moroccan Houmous and Flatbread*<br><br>• 2 clementines |
| **dinner** | | • *Sweet Potato and Chestnut Jalousie* OR<br>• *Moroccan Lamb Stew* OR<br>• *Salmon en Croûte* WITH<br>• *Orange and Mint Couscous* OR<br>• *Hot Potato Salad* AND<br>• *Watercress and Orange Salad* AND<br>• *Curly Kale with Garlic Cherry Tomatoes*<br><br>• *Traditional Rice Pudding* | • *Crab Linguine* OR<br>• *Mushroom and Asparagus Omelet* OR<br>• *Mushroom-Stuffed Chicken with Green Lentils* WITH<br>• mashed potatoes AND<br>• Peas and carrots OR<br>• *Green Beans with Chorizo*<br><br>• *Raspberry and Pomegranate Gelatin* OR<br>• *Apple and Black Currant Oat Crisp* | • *Teriyaki Turkey with Sesame Cucumber Salad* OR<br>• *Tuna Steak with Tomato Crust and Lime Dressing* OR<br>• *Tarka Dhal* WITH<br>• *Almond Rice* AND<br>• *Spinach with Dried Currants and Pine Nuts* OR<br>• *Watercress and Orange Salad*<br><br>• *Pear in Chocolate Sauce* OR<br>• 2 scoops ice cream |
| **snacks** | | • Berry smoothie<br>• *Chocolate Brazil Brownie* | • Fruit yogurt<br>• *Fruity Oat Bar* | • Fruit yogurt |

**DRINKS:** 1¼ cups low-fat milk or fortified soy equivalent in drinks throughout the day. Water ad lib throughout the day, and herb tea, coffee, and tea as guided by chapter 3. Fruit juice assumed to be 7 to 8 fl oz glass unsweetened.

| Thursday | Friday | Saturday | Sunday |
|---|---|---|---|
| • Tropical smoothie with dried fruit bread OR<br>• Oat and wheat flakes with dried fruit OR<br>• 2 hot cross buns | • *Mexican Brunch* OR<br>• Boiled eggs with whole-wheat toast OR<br>• Oat and wheat flakes with dried fruit<br><br>• Orange juice | • *Orange Bran Muffin* WITH<br>• milk OR<br>• Weetabix with raisins OR<br>• *Mushroom and Asparagus Omelet* | • Bran flakes with dried apricots OR<br>• 2 slices whole-wheat toast WITH chopped banana OR<br>• Croissant or crescent roll and preserves WITH<br>• 2 clementines |
| • *Barley and Roasted Vegetable Salad* OR<br>• *Crab Cakes with Watercress and Orange Salad*<br><br>• Fresh mango AND<br>• *Fruity Oat Bar* | • *Beef and Beet Sandwich* OR<br>• *Red Pepper Paté* WITH toast and salad AND<br>• 1 oz bag roasted vegetable chips | • *Romaine, Chicken, and Croutons* OR<br>• *Crab Cakes with Watercress and Orange Salad* OR<br>• *Baba Ganoush with Bread and Asparagus Tips*<br><br>• Fruit yogurt | • *Beef and Beet Sandwich* OR<br>• *Brazil Nut Burger* in a bun OR<br>• *Grilled Srdine and Cheese Sandwich* |
| • *Pea and Spinach Soup* AND<br>• *Chinese Beef and Noodles* OR<br>• *Jambalaya* OR<br>• *Wild Rice Pilaf with Fish. Peas, and Capers*<br><br>• Fruit yogurt | • *Brazil Nut Burgers* in a bun OR<br>• *Tarka Dhal* WITH naan OR<br>• *Paella* WITH<br>• *Broccoli and Almonds* OR<br>• *Curly Kale with Garlic Cherry Tomatoes*<br><br>• Greek yogurt WITH strawberries and honey OR<br>• *Chocolate Brioche Pudding* | • *Pork with Plums* OR<br>• *Tuna Steak with Sun-Dried Tomato Crust and Lime Dressing* OR<br>• *Creamy Vegetarian Ground "Beef"* WITH<br>• Almond rice AND<br>• *Green Chile Edamame* OR<br>• *Ginger and Orange Slaw*<br><br>• *Honey and Pistachio Fig with Yogurt* OR<br>• *Mango and Lime Dessert* | • *Crab Cake with Watercress and Orange Salad* OR<br>• *Sesame Chicken with Mango Salsa* OR<br>• *Stuffed Portobello Mushrooms* WITH<br>• *Quinoa and Sunflower Seeds* OR<br>• *Leek Potatoes* AND<br>• *Curly Kale with Garlic Cherry Tomatoes* OR<br>• Green salad with dressing<br><br>• *Raisin and Apple Pancake* OR<br>• Greek yogurt with blueberries and honey |
| • *Chocolate Brazil Brownie* | • 3 to 4 chocolate Brazil nuts | • *Cheddar and Sun-Dried Tomato Biscuit* | • *Carrot Sheet Cake* OR<br>• *Summer Fruit Compote* and ice cream |

NOTES: Portion of vegetables or fruit is 3 oz or more unless specified. Where lower fat options exist, assume these are used. All spread assumed to be reduced fat (60%) olive spread. Yogurt is low fat unless stated. Mayonnaise is 3% fat and only 1 tablespoon is used in sandwiches. Bread is an average slice of 1 oz, 2 slices per sandwich. Salad dressing is assumed to be 1 tablespoon standard French dressing.

# CHAPTER 5

# RECIPES

# citrus salad bowl

Vitamin C is vital in protecting you and your baby from infection. Citrus fruits and kiwi are among the highest providers of this vitamin and make a colorful breakfast salad.

serves  2
preparation time  5 minutes
cooking time  0 minutes

*1 medium grapefruit, color of your choice*
*2 seedless clementines*
*1 large or 2 small kiwifruit*

1 Peel the grapefruit with a sharp knife, then, holding the fruit over a mixing bowl to catch any juice, cut away each section from the membrane. Add to the bowl.
2 Peel the clementines, separate into sections, and add to the bowl.
3 Peel the kiwifruit and cut into rounds. Stir into the bowl and serve the fruit salad immediately.

### serving suggestions
*Top with toasted almonds or seeds as well as yogurt, and follow with toast, muffins, or oatmeal.*

### storage
*The fruit salad can be stored for 24 hours in an airtight container in the refrigerator, but it is not suitable for freezing.*

# raspberry oatmeal with walnuts

Oats promote heart health and are also great for keeping hunger at bay, and this hot breakfast will keep you going all morning.

serves  1
preparation time  2 minutes
cooking time  5 minutes

*½ cup rolled oats*
*1 cup lowfat milk*
*1 tablespoon maple syrup*
*3 walnut halves*

1 Put the oats and milk into a small saucepan and bring to simmering point, stirring frequently.
2 Once it has thickened, remove from the heat and add the raspberries. Let stand for a few seconds before stirring in the berries, then pour the oatmeal into a serving dish.
3 Top with the maple syrup and walnuts.

### serving suggestions
*Eat with a hot drink or a glass of fruit juice.*

### allergens
*Gluten (oats), milk, nuts (walnuts).*

**COOK'S TIP**
*Frozen raspberries are much cheaper than fresh and quickly defrost in the oatmeal.*

# raisin and apple pancakes

For a change of pace from toast and jelly, you can make these fruity pancakes. They make a great weekend brunch when you may have a little more time to cook, and there will be some leftovers to freeze for other, more rushed, mornings. Nutritionally, they provide bone-building magnesium and calcium, the B vitamins, and zinc, as well as one fifth of your iron needs.

serves  4
preparation time   10 minutes
cooking time   15 to 20 minutes

*1 cup whole wheat flour*
*1 cup white all-purpose flour*
*1 tablespoon baking powder*
*1 teaspoon ground cinnamon*
*2 large eggs*
*1 cup lowfat milk*
*2 tablespoons maple syrup*
*1 medium cooking apple*
*  (you need about ¾ cup grated apple)*
*½ cup raisins*

*Canola oil for cooking*
*Plain yogurt, to serve*

1 Preheat your oven to 225°F.
2 Sift the flours, baking powder, and cinnamon into a large mixing bowl, adding in any bran that remains.
3 Add the eggs, milk, and syrup and, using a handheld mixer or blender, combine to make a thick batter.
4 Peel the apple and grate coarsely, and add about ¾ cup of apple to the batter along with the raisins. Stir well to combine.
5 Using a medium-to-high flame or burner setting, heat a flat griddle or nonstick skillet until hot and add half a teaspoon of oil.
6 Pour a ladleful of batter onto the griddle and let spread. When it is just golden brown on the bottom, carefully turn it over with a spatula and cook on the other side. This will probably take 2 to 3 minutes per side, depending on your stove. The thicker the mixture, the lower the heat should be to make sure the inside is cooked.

7 Once the pancake is ready, remove from the pan and keep warm in the oven while you cook the remaining batter. Or, if you are keeping some for another day, let cool.
8 Serve the pancakes while still warm.

## serving suggestions
*Accompany each pancake with 1 tablespoon plain yogurt. You could also try a spoonful of maple syrup, fresh fruit, or* Summer Fruit Compote, *page 142.*

## storage
*The pancakes are ideal for freezing, so when you have made a batch, using interleaving sheets or wax paper to keep separate, and place in an airtight container. Freeze for up to 3 months. You can remove individual pancakes and defrost and reheat in a microwave cooker.*

## allergens
*Gluten (wheat ), eggs, milk (milk and yogurt).*

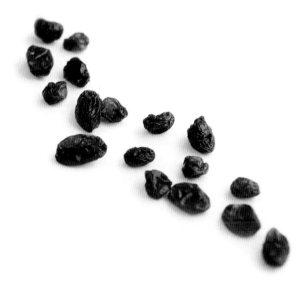

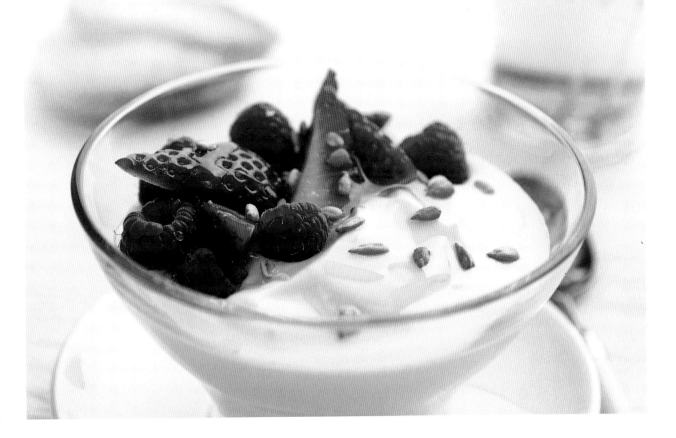

# berry yogurt breakfast

Make this colorful berry dish a regular part of your morning, because it provides all your day's vitamin C and 40 percent of your calcium requirements. The sunflower seeds also provide protective zinc and vitamin E.

serves  1
preparation time  5 minutes
cooking time  0 minutes

2/3 cup fat-free plain yogurt
1/3 cup hulled and halved strawberries
1/2 cup raspberries
1 tablespoon honey
1 tablespoon sunflower seeds, toasted

1 Spoon the yogurt into the serving bowl and top with the fruit.
2 Drizzle with the honey and then sprinkle the seeds on top.

**serving suggestions**
*Follow with a whole-wheat English muffin and a glass of juice.*

**storage**
*This is not suitable for storage.*

**allergens**
*Milk (yogurt).*

breakfasts

# Mexican brunch

Not only tasty and filling, this Mexican-style dish provides one quarter of your day's need for iron, vitamin C, and folic acid as well as being a source of fiber. So dig in, safe in the knowledge you and your baby are being well-nourished!

serves  1
preparation time  15 minutes
cooking time  15 minutes

### for the tomato salsa
*1 large ripe tomato at room temperature*
*1 tablespoon tomato chutney or relish*
*1 teaspoon chopped cilantro (optional)*

### for the scrambled eggs
*1 large egg*
*2 tablespoons lowfat milk*
*black pepper (optional)*
*1 teaspoon reduced-fat polyunsaturated spread*

*2 heaping tablespoons cooked black beans*
  *(see box right)*
*1 corn or whole-wheat tortilla wrap*

1 Preheat your oven to 225°F and place a plate in it to warm along with the tortilla wrapped in aluminum foil.
2 Cut the tomato into small pieces and mix with the chutney or relish and cilantro, if used.
3 Beat the egg it in a small bowl with the milk and pepper. Melt the spread in a small saucepan and pour in the egg mixture. Cook over low heat, stirring frequently until the egg just sets.
4 Meanwhile, heat the beans in a small saucepan, adding a little water to prevent sticking, if required.
5 Remove the tortilla and warm plate from the oven and serve the beans, salsa, and egg with the tortilla.

### serving suggestions
*Accompany with a glass of fruit juice or a smoothie.*

### allergens
*Gluten (wheat), egg, milk.*

### COOK'S TIP
*Look out for cans of black beans (sometimes called turtle beans) in water in supermarkets. Alternatively, buy dried black beans. It is worth preparing at least 1½ cups of dried beans at a time, because the cooked beans will freeze well for up to 3 months. Simply soak the dried beans overnight and then cook according to package directions.*

# mushroom and asparagus omelet

Whether you prefer something special for Sunday brunch or want a quick dinner or tasty lunch, this omelet checks many of your nutritional requirement boxes, as well as tastes great. Just make sure to cook the eggs until they are firm, putting it under a hot broiler, if necessary, to set the top.

serves 2
preparation time 10 minutes
cooking time 10 minutes

1 tablespoon vegetable oil
7 oz closed cup mushrooms, sliced
7 oz fresh asparagus
4 extra large eggs
pinch salt and little black pepper
1 teaspoon vegetable oil

1 Heat the oil in a nonstick skillet and gently sauté the mushrooms, stirring often, for 3 to 4 minutes. Cover.
2 Meanwhile, slice off the bottom ¾ inch of the asparagus stems and discard. Then cut off the tip along with about 2 inches of each stem, and place on one side. Slice the remaining stem into ¾ inch pieces, and cook with the mushrooms four about 10 minutes, until just tender.
3 While the mushrooms cook, steam the remaining asparagus tips until just tender, using a basket steamer, a saucepan (see page 80), or purpose-made asparagus steamer.
4 Beat the eggs with the seasoning and 1 tablespoon water.
5 Heat the oil in a nonstick omelet pan over medium heat and pour in the eggs. When the bottom is beginning to set, move it to the center, letting the runny egg spread to the edges. Repeat once or twice until the egg is set.
6 Fill the set omelet with the mushroom filling, slide carefully onto a warm plate, and cut in half.
7 Serve each half with half the asparagus tips on the side.

serving suggestions
*Accompany with fresh crusty bread, and a few cherry tomatoes.*

allergens
*Eggs.*

<mushroom and asparagus omelet

# baba ganoush with bread and asparagus tips

This eggplant dip is found in many countries in the Middle East, and is simple to make. Served with folate-rich asparagus tips and some whole wheat pita bread, it makes a delicious snack that provides more than one quarter of your pregnancy needs for iron, zinc, and folate. Or, you can make a meal of it by serving alongside some broiled lamb chops and Tzatziki (see page 63).

serves 2
preparation time 10 minutes
cooking time 25 minutes

1 medium eggplant
1 tablespoon tahini paste
1 clove garlic, crushed
2 teaspoons lemon juice
1 tablespoon flat leaf parsley, chopped
black pepper

**to serve**
3½ oz asparagus tips, lightly steamed
2 whole wheat pita bread, toasted

1 Preheat the broiler to high, and the oven to 400°F.
2 Cut the eggplant in half and place flesh side down under the broiler until the skin starts to blacken.
3 Remove and put into the oven until the flesh is tender—10 to 20 minutes, depending on how well broiled the eggplant was. Let cool.
4 Scoop out the flesh from the eggplant halves and place in a small bowl or blender bowl.
5 Add the tahini, garlic, and lemon juice and blend until smooth.
6 Quickly blend in the parsley and black pepper.
7 Serve with the steamed asparagus and whole wheat pita bread.

**storage**
*Baba ganoush can be stored in the refrigerator for up to 48 hours but is not suitable for freezing.*

**allergens**
*Wheat (gluten), sesame.*

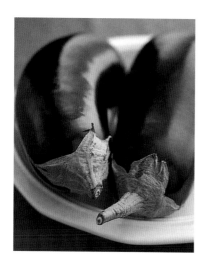

# green beans and chorizo

This supremely simple dish based on a Spanish tapa uses spicy chorizo (best bought in a block from the deli), but you could use salami if you prefer. It is rich in energy-releasing vitamin $B_1$, as well as zinc and vitamin $B_{12}$—both essential pregnancy nutrients.

serves 2
preparation time 5 minutes
cooking time 5 to 10 minutes

9½ oz stringless flat green beans, such as helda or runner beans, cut into 1 inch pieces (about 1½ cups)
3½ oz chorizo, cut into small cubes
1 tablespoon olive oil mixed with 1 tablespoon lemon juice

1 Steam the beans until just tender.
2 Cook the chorizo in a dry skillet, letting the juices flow out.
3 Add the chorizo to the beans and mix, then stir in the olive oil and lemon juice.

## serving suggestions
Eat with crusty bread or another tapas-style dish, such as Patatas Bravas, page 60.

## allergens
Chorizo may contain milk, sulfites, and wheat.

# bruschettas

The classic topping for these snacks is fresh tomatoes, but there are many variations you can make, which will not only provide interest but will boost some key pregnancy nutrients. The smoked mackerel, ricotta, and beet version makes a really healthy and colorful lunch or snack, because it provides omega 3 fatty acids and vitamins D and B$_{12}$.

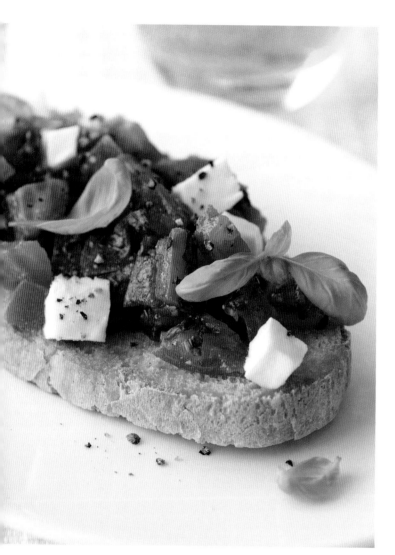

## tomato, basil, and mozzarella

serves 2
preparation time 5 minutes
cooking time 2 to 3 minutes

2 medium tomatoes, quartered and seeds removed
pinch salt
black pepper
2 to 3 large basil leaves, coarsely torn
1 tablespoon olive oil
2 slices bruschettina or 2 (¾ inch) slices of a large ciabatta
1 clove garlic, peeled
2 oz fresh mozzarella, cut into cubes

1 Coarsely chop the tomatoes, and mix with the salt, pepper, basil, and olive oil. Let infuse for a few minutes.
2 Meanwhile, toast the bruschettina and scrape the garlic clove over the bread.
3 Spoon the topping over the bread and add a the cubes of mozzarella.

### allergens
*Wheat (gluten) , milk (mozzarella).*

## STORAGE
*The completed bruschettas should be eaten immediately, but each of the toppings can be kept in the refrigerator for up to 24 hours.*

## roasted pepper and olive

serves 2
preparation time  5 minutes
cooking time  30 minutes

---

½ medium red and ½ medium green bell pepper, cut into large chunks
2 teaspoons olive oil
2 slices bruschettina or 2 (¾ inch) slices of a large ciabatta
⅓ cup sliced, drained pitted black olives in liquid
2 teaspoons tomato paste

1 Preheat an oven to 400°F.
2 Put the bell peppers into a small roasting or ovenproof dish and drizzle with the oil.
3 Roast for 25 to 30 minutes, turning occasionally to coat in the oil, until the bell peppers are softened.
4 Let cool, and chop coarsely into smaller pieces.
5 Lightly toast the bread and spread each slice with the tomato paste.
6 Mix the peppers with the black olives and spoon on to the bread.

allergens
*Wheat (gluten).*

## smoked mackerel, ricotta, and beets

serves 3
preparation time  15 minutes
cooking time  2 to 3 minutes

---

1 fillet smoked mackerel (around 2¾ oz)
1 tablespoon lemon juice
2 oz ricotta
1 teaspoon hot horseradish
1 tablespoon parsley, finely chopped
1 cooked beet, coarsely chopped
3 slices bruschettina or 3 (¾ inch) slices of a large ciabatta
olive oil

1 Remove the skin from the mackerel and discard.
2 Put the mackerel and lemon juice into a mixing bowl and using a fork, break up the fish.
3 Add the ricotta, horseradish, and parsley and mix until smooth.
4 Mix in the cooked beet.
5 Meanwhile, toast the bread and drizzle with a little olive oil. Top with the fish mixture.

allergens
*Wheat (gluten), milk (ricotta).*

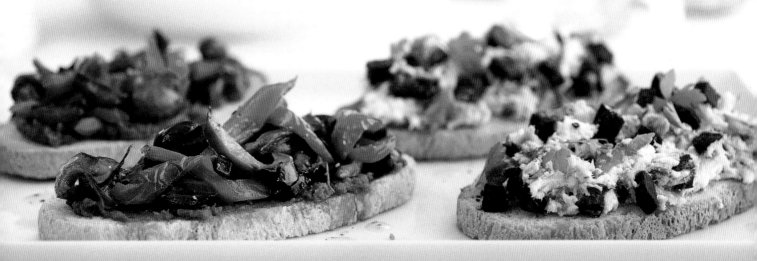

# patatas bravas

Even taking into account nutrients lost through cooking, this dish is rich in vitamin C, and it is simple to make. The tomato sauce is a pregnancy basic, so it's well worth making double the quantity you need and freezing half. It can then be used to accompany meat, chicken, or fish, or served with pasta.

serves  4 as an appetizer
preparation time  15 minutes
cooking time  40 to 50 minutes

**for the potatoes**
*1½ lb roasting potatoes, such as russets, scrubbed and cut into ¾ inch cubes*
*2 tablespoons vegetable oil*

**for the tomato sauce**
*1 tablespoon olive oil*
*1 medium onion, finely chopped*
*2 cloves garlic, crushed*
*1 teaspoon paprika (optional)*
*1 teaspoon chili powder (optional)*
*2⅔ cups canned diced tomatoes in tomato juice*
*2 tablespoons tomato paste*
*pinch sugar*
*black pepper*

**to serve**
*2 tablespoons parsley, chopped*

**COOK'S TIP**
*There's no need to peel the potatoes, just make sure they are well scrubbed.*

1 Preheat the oven to 400°F.
2 Put the oil into a roasting pan and heat in the oven until hot.
3 Add the potatoes and turn them to coat in the oil.
4 Roast the potatoes, turning occasionally, for 40 to 50 minutes, until golden and crisp.
5 Meanwhile, prepare the sauce by heating the oil in a nonstick saucepan and sautéing the onion until softened.
6 Add the garlic, spices, if using, canned tomatoes, and tomato paste, and stir in the sugar.
7 Bring to a boil, stirring, and then simmer for 10 to 15 minutes, until the sauce is pulpy and soft.
8 Season to taste with black pepper.
9 When the potatoes are cooked, place in a serving dish and cover with the sauce. Sprinkle with the chopped parsley.

**serving suggestions**
*Eat with other little plates as part of a tapas-style meal or as an accompaniment to a main-dish course.*

**storage**
*The sauce can be stored in an airtight container in the refrigerator for up to 48 hours. Alternatively, the sauce can be frozen and reheated until piping hot.*

**VARIATION**
*Omit the spices from the sauce and add your favorite herbs, or drop in a few black olives and some lemon zest, or add some chopped red or yellow bell pepper.*

little bites

# mediterranean vegetable packages

Just one of these tasty packages provides half of the vitamin C you need each day in pregnancy, but you may well be tempted to eat two as a main dish. Just add some couscous or tabbouleh and a tomato salad for a great meal.

serves 4
preparation time   10 minutes
cooking time   25 minutes

1 medium zucchini
½ medium red bell pepper
½ medium yellow bell pepper
1 small red onion, finely chopped
1 tablespoon oregano, freshly chopped
1 tablespoon mint, freshly chopped
3½ oz feta cheese, cut into cubes
black pepper
8 sheets phyllo pastry
2 tablespoon vegetable oil

1 Preheat the oven to 400°F.
2 Cut the zucchini and bell peppers into ¾ inch dice and put into a bowl. Add the chopped onion and herbs and mix well.
3 Add the feta and grind some black pepper over the top.
4 Place the phyllo pastry on a board and brush or spray the top piece with oil.
5 Spoon one quarter of the vegetable mixture into the center and wrap to make a rectangular package.
6 Brush another sheet with oil and wrap the package again, this time placing the thicker layer on top. Place on to a baking sheet lined with nonstick parchment paper.
7 Make another three packages.
8 Lightly brush or spray the finished packages with oil and bake for 25 minutes or until golden brown.

### serving suggestions
*The packages can be eaten hot or at room temperature accompanied by a side salad and some bread, or by Tabbouleh with Pine Nuts, page 64.*

### storage
*For maximum vitamin C content, serve these packages on the day they are made, but they can be stored in the refrigerator for up to 48 hours and reheated until piping hot.*

### allergens
*Wheat (gluten), milk (feta cheese).*

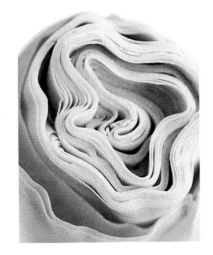

### VARIATION
*Use finely chopped eggplant, cherry tomatoes, and a few olives or capers instead of the zucchini or bell peppers.*

# roasted red pepper pâté

This delicious vegetarian pâté is not only full of finely flavored ingredients, but it's a wonderful way of getting plenty of vitamins C and A. It makes a great lunch with crusty bread and a mixed salad, or can be served alongside some of the other little dishes in this section.

serves  4
preparation time  10 minutes
cooking time  30 minutes

2 red bell peppers, cut into large chunks
½ red onion, peeled and chopped
2 tablespoons olive oil
5 large fresh basil leaves, torn into 2 or 3 pieces
1 clove garlic, peeled and chopped
3½ oz mascarpone cheese
1 teaspoon tomato paste
2 teaspoons lemon juice
black pepper, to taste

1 Preheat the oven to 200°F.
2 Put the bell peppers and onion into a roasting pan, drizzle with the oil, and roast in the oven for 30 minutes, or until the bell peppers are soft.
3 Let cool for a few minutes, then transfer the mixture to a food processor. Add the basil and pulse lightly to mix. Add the remaining ingredients and pulse again until smooth.
4 Spoon the pâté into individual ramekins or one large dish. Chill before serving.

### serving suggestions
*Eat on toasted walnut or seed bread alongside a crisp green salad.*

### storage
*The pâté can be stored in an airtight container in the refrigerator for up to 48 hours but is not suitable for freezing.*

### allergens
*Milk.*

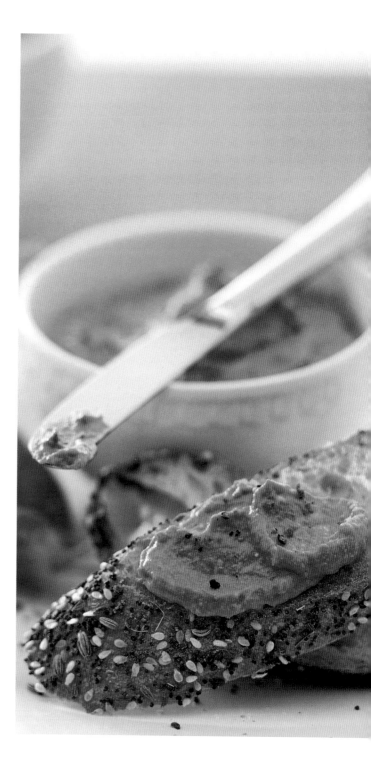

little bites

# tzatziki with raw vegetables

It's not so much the dip, but the vegetables that give this simple snack its high nutritional value. Cauliflower, baby corn, and carrot provide essential vitamins A, C, and folate, and because they are eaten raw, cooking losses are vastly reduced. The Greek yogurt also contains valuable calcium and riboflavin and the quantities are similar whether you choose 0-percent fat yogurt as specified, or go for one that has a 2-percent fat content.

serves 2
preparation time 20 minutes

2¾ inch piece of cucumber
salt
⅔ cup fat-free Greek yogurt
1 tablespoon extra virgin olive oil
1 tablespoon mint, chopped
1 medium carrot, scrubbed and sliced into batons
2 florets cauliflower, cut into smaller pieces
3–4 baby corn, washed and steamed, if you prefer

**optional extras**
1 clove garlic, crushed
Zest of 1 lemon
Dill, to replace mint, if preferred

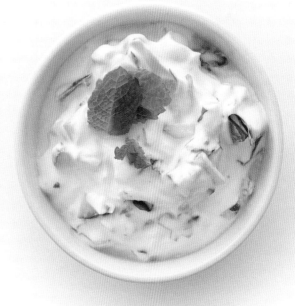

1 Wash the cucumber and slice lengthwise. Scoop out the seeds, then chop into small pieces.
2 Place in a colander or on some paper towels and sprinkle with a pinch or two of salt. Let stand for 10 to 15 minutes until some water drains from the cucumber.
3 Meanwhile, mix the yogurt with the oil and mint.
4 Pat dry the cucumber, wiping away any excess salt, and mix into the yogurt.
5 Serve immediately, with the vegetables.

**serving suggestions**
*This makes a great accompaniment to lamb chops or other broiled meat, or poultry.*

**storage**
*Tzatziki can be stored in the refrigerator for up to 24 hours but is not suitable for freezing.*

**allergens**
*Milk (yogurt).*

little bites

# moroccan hummus with flatbread

- - - - - - - - - - - - - - - -

This simple dip, if eaten with whole wheat pita bread, meets one quarter of your daily requirements for iron and one third for zinc.

- - - - - - - - - - - - - - - - - - - - - - - - - - - -

serves  4
preparation time  5 minutes
cooking time  0 minutes

- - - - - - - - - - - - - - - - - - - - - - - - - - - -

1 2/3 cups drained, canned chickpeas in water
1 heaping tablespoon tahini paste
juice of 1 lime or ½ lemon
1 clove garlic
1 teaspoon harissa paste or Moroccan spice paste (ras el hanout)
1 to 2 tablespoons olive oil
about ¼ cup water
whole wheat pita bread or breadsticks

1 Put all the ingredients into a food processor or blender and blend until smooth, adding enough water to make a smooth pastelike consistency.
2 Chill for at least 30 minutes before serving.

### serving suggestions
Eat with and strips of bell peppers, carrots, cucumber, and celery.

### storage
The hummus can be stored in the refrigerator for up to 48 hours but is not suitable for freezing.

### allergens
Sesame; pita bread contains wheat (gluten).

# tabbouleh with pine nuts

- - - - - - - - - - - -

This great little dish is a surprising source of iron and zinc as well as vitamin E—all of which your baby needs to grow and develop.

- - - - - - - - - - - - - - - - - - - - - - - - - - - -

serves  3
preparation time  10 minutes
cooking time  15 minutes

- - - - - - - - - - - - - - - - - - - - - - - - - - - -

1 heaping cup mixed quinoa and bulgur wheat, or ½ heaping cup of each
2 medium tomatoes, seeds removed, diced
2¾ inch cucumber, cut into small dice
½ avocado, diced, tossed in 1 teaspoon lime juice
1 tablespoon mint, chopped
1 tablespoon parsley, chopped
black pepper, to taste
⅓ cup pine nuts, toasted

1 Cook the quinoa and bulgur wheat according to the package directions.
2 Drain and let cool slightly.
3 Mix in the tomatoes, cucumber, avocado, and herbs and grind some black pepper over the top.
4 Serve, sprinkled with the pine nuts.

### serving suggestions
Eat as an accompaniment to broiled meat or poultry or alongside the Mediterranean Vegetable Packages, page 61.

### storage
Tabbouleh is best served freshly made to preserve its vitamin content, but it can be stored in the refrigerator for up to 24 hours.

### allergens
Wheat (gluten), pine nuts.

# sardine and red pepper strudels

This delicious, simple recipe packs in a lot of baby-friendly nutrients per mouthful. As well as calcium, you'll be enjoying omega 3 fatty acids, vitamin $B_{12}$, and vitamin D, all of which are baby body-building essentials. If you're not usually a sardine fan, just try this, and you may be surprised just how good it tastes.

serves 2
preparation time 15 minutes
cooking time 15 minutes

2 sheets phyllo pastry (about 3½ oz)
oil mister
4 canned sardines in oil, drained
1 tablespoon lemon juice
½ red bell pepper, finely sliced
2 teaspoons fresh cilantro, chopped
grated zest of ½ lemon
black pepper, to taste

1 Preheat the oven to 400°F.
2 Place one sheet of phyllo pastry on a clean, dry work surface or cutting board and spray with a little oil.
3 Place 2 of the sardines on the pastry and top with half of the lemon juice, sliced bell pepper, cilantro, and lemon zest. Season with a little black pepper.
4 Roll up the pastry, tucking the ends under, and place on a lightly oiled baking sheet or one lined with parchment paper. Repeat steps 2 through 4 to make the second package. Spray the packages with some more oil and bake for 15 minutes or until golden.

## serving suggestions
Garnish with sliced lemon and eat with a salad of mixed greens and sliced fresh tomatoes.

## storage
The strudel can be kept in an airtight container in the refrigerator for up to 24 hours but is not suitable for freezing. Reheat until piping hot.

## allergens
Wheat (gluten), fish.

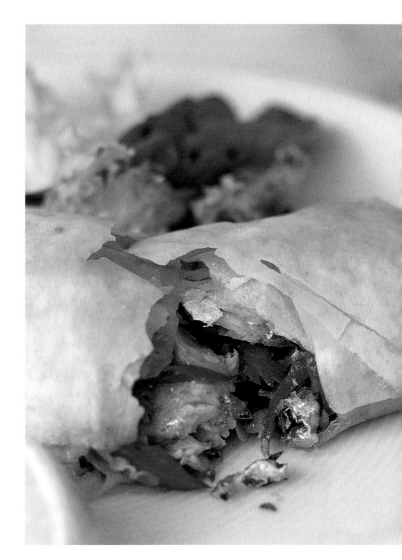

## VARIATION
If you prefer, use sardines in tomato sauce, or canned mackerel; canned tuna isn't such a nutritious substitute.

little bites

# homemade fish sticks
# with piquant avocado dip

Use your favorite sustainable white fish, such as halibut, red snapper, cod, sole, or catfish, to make these fish sticks. Serving them with the piquant dip will meet more than 50 percent of your pregnancy requirement for vitamin B$_{12}$, and provides more than one quarter of the calcium and magnesium your baby needs for her bones and teeth.

serves  2 to 3
preparation time  15 minutes
cooking time  15 minutes

*2 white fish fillets (8–9 oz)*
*2 slices whole-grain bread made into bread crumbs*
  *or ½ cup dried bread crumbs*
*zest of ½ lime, finely grated*
*black pepper*
*1 medium egg, beaten*

**for the piquant avocado dip**
*½ avocado, cut into small cubes*
*zest of ½ lime, finely grated*
*1 teaspoon lime juice*
*2 tablespoons finely chopped cornichons*
  *(small pickles)*
*¾ cup Greek yogurt*
*black pepper*

1 Preheat the oven to 400°F.
2 Cut the fish fillets into strips around ¾ inch wide.
3 Mix the bread crumbs with the lime zest and black pepper and spoon onto a plate.
4 Line a baking sheet with parchment paper.
5 Pour the well-beaten egg into a shallow dish.
6 Carefully dip each strip of fish into the egg and coat well, then transfer to the bread crumbs. Spoon the crumbs over the fish and press lightly so they adhere. Carefully lift the fish onto the baking sheet.
7 Bake the fish for 10 to 15 minutes or until crispy. Test one piece of fish; it should be easy to break. Set the fish aside while you make the dip.
8 Combine the cubes of avocado with the lime zest and juice. Stir in the cornichons and yogurt and season with black pepper.

**serving suggestions**
Eat the fish hot with the dip *on its own alongside other small plates, such as Patatas Bravas, page 60, or Tabbouleh with Pine Nuts, page 64.*

**storage**
*Both the fish sticks and dip are best served immediately, but the dip can be stored in the refrigerator for up to 24 hours.*

**allergens**
*Wheat (gluten), eggs, fish.*

<piquant avocado dip

# ratatouille with cheese and bread

A stew made from bell peppers, zucchini, eggplant, tomatoes, and onion, known as ratatouille in France, makes a delicious side dish or accompanied by lightly fried halloumi cheese (available in Middle Eastern or gourmet stores) and pita bread, can be eaten as a simple lunch or substantial appetizer that provides vitamins A and C, as well as a range of different flavors and textures. If you've never tried halloumi before, be prepared to be enticed by its great taste and versatility in cooking—fried or broiled it shines. It is, however, high in salt, so don't go overboard.

serves 4
preparation time 15 minutes
cooking time 45 to 50 minutes

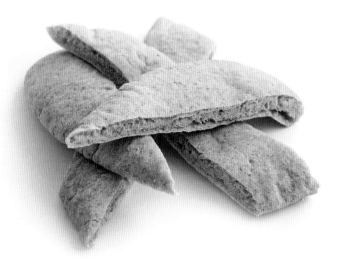

### for the ratatouille
*1 tablespoon olive oil*
*1 medium onion, sliced*
*2 cloves garlic, crushed*
*2 bell peppers of different colors, cut into large dice*
*1 small eggplant, cut into ¾ inch dice*
*1 medium zucchini, cut into ¾ inch dice*
*3 medium tomatoes, quartered*
*1²/₃ cups canned diced tomatoes in tomato juice*
*1 tablespoon oregano, chopped*

*9 oz haloumi or mozzarella cheese, sliced*
*1 tablespoon olive oil*
*4 pita bread*

1 Heat 1 tablespoon olive oil in a large ovenproof casserole and sauté the onion and garlic for 3 to 4 minutes.
2 Add the bell peppers, eggplant, and zucchini and stir over medium heat for 5 minutes.
3 Stir in the fresh and canned tomatoes and oregano.
4 Cover and cook over low heat stirring occasionally, for 40 to 45 minutes, or cook in an oven at 350°F for the same amount of time.
6 Meanwhile, heat 1 tablespoon olive oil and cook the halloumi until golden on one side, then turn and cook the other side similarly.
7 Lightly toast the pita bread and slice into strips.
8 Serve the ratatouille hot with the haloumi and pita bread strips alongside.

### serving suggestions
*The ratatouille on its own makes a tasty accompaniment to steak, broiled chicken, or fish and will serve 4 to 6. After cooking, add 1 tablespoon chopped parsley and a few basil leaves, torn coarsely.*

### storage
*The ratatouille can be stored in the refrigerator for up to 48 hours though it will lose some of its vitamin C content. It can also be frozen for up to 3 months and reheated until piping hot.*

### allergens
*Wheat (gluten), milk (halloumi).*

little bites

# bean and salsa wrap

For an easy way to boost your fiber intak,e tuck some spinach leaves, grated cheese, and warmed refried beans into a wrap. This will provide you with half your daily requirements for vitamin A and calcium, too.

serves  1
preparation time  5 minutes
cooking time  2 minutes

*1 seeded or whole wheat tortilla wrap, warmed*
*½ small can (7½ oz) refried beans, warmed*
*1 tablespoon tomato salsa or relish*
*1 cup baby spinach leaves*
*¼ cup shredded reduced-fat cheddar cheese*

1 Spread the warmed beans over the wrap and add the salsa.
2 Sprinkle with the cheese and spinach leaves.
3 Roll up the wrap and cut in half.
4 Serve immediately.

## serving suggestions
*Serve with a few cherry tomatoes or a lowfat dip and celery crudités.*

## allergens
*Gluten (wheat), milk (cheese). Sesame if seeded wraps used.*

# beef and beet sandwich

You can make a simple, highly nutritious sandwich with roast beef, which is rich in iron. Teamed here with folate-rich beet, horseradish, and watercress you'll enjoy a superb sandwich.

serves  1
preparation time  5 minutes
cooking time  0 minutes

*1 level tablespoon creamed horseradish*
*1 level tablespoon Greek-style yogurt*
*2 medium slices whole wheat bread*
*2 oz sliced lean beef*
*1 cooked beet, sliced*
*8 sprigs of watercress*
*olive spread*

1 Mix together the horseradish and yogurt and spread over one slice of the bread.
2 Place the beef, beets, and watercress on top.
3 Spread the remaining slice with olive spread and use to make the sandwich.
4 Serve immediately.

## serving suggestions
*Serve with a few carrot sticks, and a glass of orange juice.*

## storage
*The sandwich will keep over night in the refrigerator if wrapped in plastic wrap, but is best served immediately.*

## allergens
*Gluten (wheat), milk (yogurt).*

little bites

68

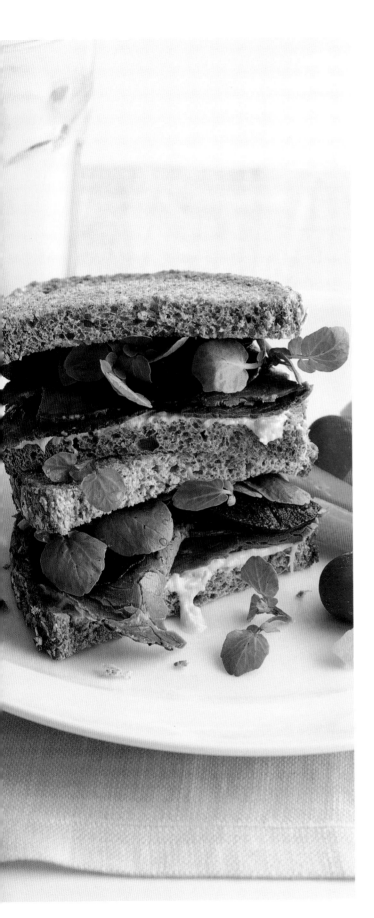

# grilled sardine and cheese sandwich

Canned sardines should be a pantry essential in pregnancy, because they are so good for you and your baby. This simple sandwich lunch meets many of your pregnancy nutrition needs, containing omega 3 fatty acids, vitamins B12 and D, calcium, iron, and zinc. In fact, you should make it a weekly lunch.

serves  1
preparation time  5 minutes
cooking time  3 to 4 minutes

*2 canned sardines in oil (about 2 oz), drained*
*1 teaspoon lemon juice*
*2 thick slices bread with added fiber*
*few slices red bell pepper*
*1 slice reduced-fat cheddar cheese*

1 Mash the sardines and lemon juice with a fork and spread over one slice of the bread.
2 Add the sliced bell pepper and top with the cheese. Add the other piece of bread to make a lid.
3 Place in a sandwich toaster until the cheese has melted and the bread is golden.
4 Serve immediately.

## serving suggestions
*Serve with a handful of salad greens or a few cherry tomatoes.*

## allergens
*Gluten (wheat), fish.*

# egg, tomato, and onion roll

This simple filled egg roll provides your baby with bone-building calcium and immune-boosting zinc as well as tastes great. Instead of regular mayonnaise, it uses a combination of yogurt and lowfat mayonnaise with scallions and tomatoes to provide a fresh tang. Use multigrain bread or rolls, because they provide more folic acid than other breads (unless they have been fortified).

serves 1
preparation time 5 minutes
cooking time 10 minutes

1 large egg
1 small tomato
1 level tablespoon lowfat plain yogurt
1 level tablespoon "lite" mayonnaise (less than
    3% fat)
2 scallions, chopped
black pepper to taste
1 large multigrain roll or 2 slices multigrain bread

1 Hard boil the egg and cool immediately in cold,
  running water.
2 Skin the tomato, remove the seeds, and chop
  coarsely.
3 Mix the yogurt and mayonnaise with the scallion
  and tomato and season with black pepper.
4 When the egg is cool enough, peel and chop into the
  mix and stir well.
5 Halve the roll and spoon the egg mixture over the
  bottom. Put on the top and eat immediately.

## serving suggestions
*Serve with a handful of arugula or watercress.*

## storage
*The sandwich could be refrigerated wrapped in plastic wrap for 24 hours, but is best served immediately. It is not suitable for freezing.*

## allergens
*Contains: gluten (wheat), eggs, milk (yogurt).*

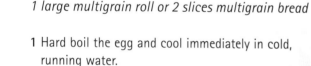

>barley and roasted vegetable salad with pumpkin seeds

little bites

# barley and roasted vegetable salad with pumpkin seeds

This high-fiber salad is an ideal way to use leftover roasted vegetables, but you can obviously start from scratch, if you prefer. Offset any vitamin losses from using leftovers by adding in fresh ingredients, in this case parsley and pomegranate seeds. The barley and pumpkin seeds also provide nearly half your day's requirement for blood and bone-building iron.

serves  1
preparation time  10 minutes
cooking time  5 minutes

3 tablespoons pumpkin seeds
½ recipe of Herbed Barley, page 137
½ recipe of Roast Beet and Butternut Squash,
    page 135
2 teaspoons freshly chopped parsley
2½ tablespoons pomegranate seeds

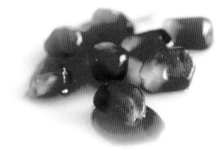

1 Toast the pumpkin seeds either in a dry skillet on the stove or in a preheated oven at 400°F until just lightly browned and crisp. Cool.
2 Meanwhile, combine the barley and roasted vegetables, and stir in the parsley.
3 Sprinkle with the pomegranate and pumpkin seeds and serve.

**serving suggestions**
*Accompany with a glass of unsweetened juice.*

**allergens**
*Gluten (barley).*

**COOK'S TIP**
*When pomegranates are out of season, use a few little ripe tomatoes, or one quarter of a chopped red bell pepper instead.*

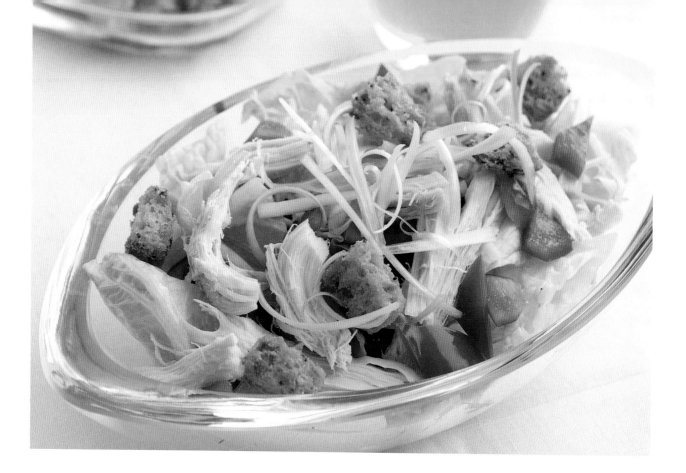

# romaine, chicken, and croutons

A lighter version than the usual fat-laden chicken Caesar salad, this dish provides the essential B vitamins to help release energy, and vitamin C for your baby's many developing cells.

serves 1
preparation time 5 minutes
cooking time 15 minutes

1 thick slice seeded bread
olive oil or other vegetable oil spray
1 heaping cup shredded romaine lettuce
¼ cup diced red bell pepper
2 scallions, cut into ¾ inch slices
⅓ cup cooked chicken breast pieces
1 tablespoon French dressing

1 Preheat the oven to 400°F.
2 Cut the bread into coarse cubes and spray with the oil. Bake for 10 to 15 minutes, until crispy.
3 Meanwhile prepare the other salad ingredients and place in a serving bowl.
4 When the croutons are ready, add to the salad and stir in the French dressing and serve immediately.

serving suggestions
*This is a complete dish, but if you are still hungry, add some more seeded bread.*

allergens
*Gluten (wheat), may contain sesame seeds in bread.*

# quinoa, feta, and spinach salad

This simple salad provides many of the pregnancy nutrition essentials as well as tastes great. It supplies iron (interestingly mostly from the quinoa rather than the spinach), calcium, zinc, as well as vitamins A, B3, and C. So enjoy it knowing you and your baby are benefitting.

serves  2
preparation time  5 minutes
cooking time  20 minutes

*¾ cup quinoa*
*2 cups baby spinach leaves*
*½ cup chopped, drained sun-dried tomatoes in oil*
*3½ oz feta cheese, cut into cubes*
*1 small zucchini, washed and diced*
*black pepper*

1 Cook the quinoa according to the package directions. Let cool.
2 Meanwhile, wash and spin dry the spinach leaves and place in two salad bowls.
3 When the quinoa is cooked and still warm, stir in the tomatoes, feta, and zucchini and season with black pepper.
4 Spoon on top of the spinach leaves and serve immediately.

### serving suggestions
*Serve with a glass of unsweetened citrus juice to aid iron absorption.*

### storage
*Once the salad has been made, it is not suitable for storage, but the cooked quinoa may be refrigerated for up to 48 hours or frozen for 2 months.*

### allergens
*Milk (cheese).*

# watercress and salmon salad

Full of immune-boosting vitamin A, watercress is a great partner for salmon, which supplies essential omega 3 fatty acids and vitamin D. For simplicity, choose poached salmon from the deli or lightly smoked chunky slices, opting for the lowest in sodium. Finish with a simple drizzle of balsamic glaze.

serves  1
preparation time  5 minutes
cooking time  0 minutes

*12 sprigs of watercress, washed and drained*
*2½ oz poached salmon*
*4 mozzarella balls, halved*
*6 to 8 cherry tomatoes, halved*
*balsamic glaze*

1 Break the watercress into small sections and place in the serving dish.
2 Flake the salmon on top, then add the tomatoes and mozzarella.
3 Drizzle with some balsamic glaze and serve immediately.

### serving suggestions
*Accompany with bread or new potatoes, or the* Hot Potato Salad, *page 138.*

### allergens
*Fish.*

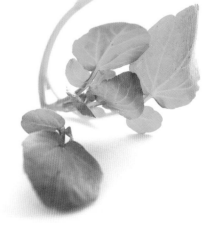

# asparagus risotto

A vegetarian risotto made with folate-rich asparagus, which will slip down easily on days when you are not feeling like eating rich food. Parmesan cheese is safe to eat in pregnancy even if it is unpasteurized.

serves 2
preparation time 5 minutes
cooking time 20 to 25 minutes

1 medium onion, finely chopped
2 tablespoons olive oil
¾ cup short-grain or risotto rice
2 tablespoons white vermouth or dry white wine
    (optional)
1¾ cups reduced-sodium vegetable broth
8 oz fine asparagus, trimmed and cut into
    ½ inch pieces
1 tablespoon finely chopped parsley
¼ cup finely grated Parmesan cheese
juice of 1 lemon
black pepper, to taste

1 Sauté the onion in the oil in a nonstick saucepan
   for 3 to 4 minutes to soften but don't brown.
2 Add the rice and stir well, then pour in the
   vermouth or dry white wine, if using, and cook
   over medium heat.
3 When the vermouth or wine has reduced, stir
   in ½ cup of the vegetable broth and allow it
   to be absorbed.
4 Then stir in another ½ cup of broth and allow it
   to be absorbed. Continue adding broth and waiting
   for it to be absorbed until all the broth is used.
5 When there is no broth left, stir in the asparagus,
   cover, and cook over medium heat for 5 minutes.
6 The risotto should now be ready, with soft rice and
   tender asparagus. Remove from the heat and stir in
   the parsley, Parmesan, and lemon juice. Check for
   seasoning, adding black pepper to taste.

**serving suggestions**
*Accompany with additional Parmesan or cheddar
cheese, and a green salad.*

**allergens**
*Milk (Parmesan).*

# Chinese beef and noodles

Rich in iron and zinc, beef is a great food for you and your baby. You can use any steak appropriate for frying in this recipe, and a 5½-ounce sirloin steak makes two generous portions along with mushrooms and noodles.

serves 2
preparation time 10 minutes
cooking time 20 minutes

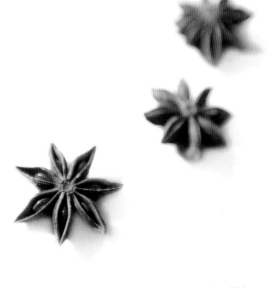

*1 tablespoon vegetable oil*
*1 small onion, sliced*
*2 cloves garlic, crushed*
*¾ inch piece ginger, grated*
*2½ cups sliced cremini mushrooms*
*1 tablespoon flour*
*1 teaspoon Chinese five spice*
*5½ oz sirloin or tenderloin steak, cut into ¾ inch wide strips*
*1 cup beef broth*
*1 tablespoon soy sauce*
*10 oz medium, straight-to-wok noodles or prepared noodles*
*5½ oz bok choy, cut in half lengthwise*

1 Heat the oil in a medium, nonstick sauté pan (one that has a lid) and sauté the onion, garlic, and ginger for 2 to 3 minutes.
2 Stir in the mushrooms and sauté for another 2 to 3 minutes, until they start to soften.
3 Meanwhile, place the flour, spice, and strips of steak in a clean, plastic food bag and shake until the steak is coated with the flour.
4 Stir the seasoned steak into the mushroom-and-onion mix and cook for 2 to 3 minutes over medium heat, turning frequently, until the steak is just brown.
5 Pour the broth and soy sauce over the mixture, stir, cover, and simmer gently until the onions and

mushrooms are just tender. There should still be plenty of fairly runny sauce, but add a little water if the sauce is too thick.
6 Now stir in the noodles, and place the bok choy on top. Cover and continue cooking over low heat for 4 to 5 minutes or until the bok choy is wilted and just tender. Serve at once in two warm bowls.

## storage
*The complete dish is not suitable for storage, but you can cook up to the end of step 5 and refrigerate the mixture for 2 days or freeze it for up to 3 months. If freezing, defrost in the refrigerator overnight, then complete the recipe from step 6.*

## allergens
*Gluten (wheat), soy.*

one-pot dishes

75

# chorizo and black-eyed peas with israeli couscous

Black-eyed peas are peculiarly rich in folate (folic acid), and are readily available in cans in the supermarket, or you can buy dried beans to soak and boil. Combined with chorizo and Israeli couscous (sometimes called pearl couscous), along with a little spinach thrown in at the last minute, gives you a highly nutritious meal for two on the table in less than 30 minutes.

serves  2
preparation time  5 to 10 minutes
cooking time  15 minutes

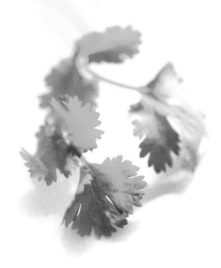

*3½ oz chorizo sausage, skin removed and cubed*
*½ onion, finely chopped*
*1 stick celery, finely sliced*
*2 cloves garlic, crushed*
*1 teaspoon ground cumin*
*1 teaspoon ground coriander*
*1 cup cooked black-eyed peas or 1 cup drained and
  rinsed canned black beans in water*
*⅓ cup Israeli couscous*
*1 cup water*
*3½ cups spinach leaves, rinsed*

1 Heat the chorizo cubes in a medium, heavy saucepan (a cast iron Dutch oven is ideal) over medium heat to release some of the fat, then stir in the onion, celery, and garlic. Cook gently until the onion is starting to soften, reducing the heat slightly if the onion starts to brown too much.
2 Stir in the spices, then add the beans, couscous, and water and bring to the boil.
3 Stir, cover, and simmer gently for 10 minutes, stirring occasionally.
4 Meanwhile place the spinach in a colander and wilt by pouring boiling water over it.
5 When the couscous is just tender, stir in the spinach and heat for another couple of minutes. Serve at once in two warm bowls.

**serving suggestions**
*Pour over a little lemon juice.*

**storage**
*This may be stored in the refrigerator for 24 hours, and reheated until piping hot. It is not suitable for freezing.*

**allergens**
*Gluten (couscous), celery, chorizo may contain wheat, milk, or sulfites.*

one-pot dishes

76

# jambalaya

This Creole dish is rich in protein and is a great source of the B vitamins, especially $B_{12}$, niacin ($B_3$), and thiamine ($B_1$). It makes a quick, nutritious dinner that minimizes dish washing and maximizes taste. Cajun spices are often salted, and the chorizo and shrimp are salty, too, so don't be tempted to add more.

serves 2
preparation time 10 minutes
cooking time 20 to 25 minutes

2½ oz chorizo bought as a piece and cubed
1 small onion, coarsely chopped
3½ oz pork tenderloin, cut into small pieces
½ small green or red bell pepper, coarsely chopped
¾ cup rice, rinsed
1 teaspoon Cajun spice
¾ cup canned diced tomatoes in juice
1¼ cups water
3½ oz cooked shrimp
1 tablespoon chopped parsley

1 Heat the chorizo in a nonstick sauté pan (one that has a lid) over low heat to release the fat. Then add the onion and cook for 5 minutes, until the onion softens, stirring occasionally.
2 Add the pork and bell peppers and turn up the heat a little. Cook for 5 minutes stirring frequently.
3 Add the rice, Cajun spice, tomatoes, and water and bring to a boil. Cover and reduce the heat and let cook for 12 to 15 minutes, until the rice is almost tender. Stir occasionally, checking to see if more water is needed and add more water, if required.
4 When the rice is just tender, stir in the cooked shrimp and heat through.
5 Spoon into two bowls and sprinkle with the parsley.

## serving suggestions
*Accompany with some small peas, which can be added to the pan along with the shrimp during the last few minutes of cooking.*

## storage
*The jambalaya will keep for 24 hours in the refrigerator but will be less rich in vitamins than when freshly cooked.*

## allergens
*Shellfish, chorizo may contain milk, wheat, and sulfites.*

# roasted pork balls and vegetables

This simple dish centers around ground pork made into balls, which are nestled into vegetables and roasted in a hot oven for a delicious meal. Pork is rich in thiamine (vitamin B$_1$), which helps to release energy from food, so this is a great meal if you are feeling a little lethargic.

serves  2
preparation time  10 minutes
cooking time  50 to 60 minutes

7½ oz waxy potatoes, such as Yukon gold, cut into wedges
1½ cups butternut squash cubes
½ red bell pepper, cut into wide strips
1 small red onion, cut into wedges
5–6 cherry tomatoes
2 tablespoons olive oil
7½ oz lean ground pork
1 slice white bread, ripped into several pieces
1 clove garlic
few sage leaves or 1 teaspoon dried sage
1 to 2 teaspoons Cajun seasoning (optional) or black pepper

1 Preheat the oven to 400°F.
2 To evenly coat the vegetables with oil, place all the vegetables in a clean plastic food bag and pour in the olive oil. Shake to coat, then transfer the vegetables to a 10 x 10 inch roasting pan.
3 Place the pork, bread, garlic, and sage in a blender or food processor and process until mixed together. Shape into 8 even balls, and tuck them in among the vegetables.
4 If you like Cajun seasoning, sprinkle it over all the ingredients. Alternatively, use a little black pepper.
5 Place the pan in the oven and cook until golden brown. After 20 to 25 minutes, remove the pan from the oven and turn over the vegetables and pork balls. Replace and continue cooking for the suggested time or until the pork balls and potatoes are golden.
6 Serve immediately.

serving suggestions
*Accompany with a prepared salsa or a lowfat sour cream dip if you have used Cajun seasoning or with Apple, Sage, and Walnut Sauce, page 104.*

allergens
*Gluten (bread).*

# sausage and orzo stew

Quick, filling, and full of vital iron and vitamin C, this simple stew uses sausages of your choice, and cooks in less than half a hour.

serves  2
preparation time  5 minutes
cooking time  20 to 25 minutes

*3–4 premium link sausages of your choice*
  *(about 7½ oz)*
*1 medium onion, finely chopped*
*1 tablespoon vegetable oil*
*1 (14½ oz) can diced tomatoes in juice*
*¾ cup orzo*
*1 cup chicken broth*
*1 teaspoon oregano*
*3½ cups baby spinach leaves*

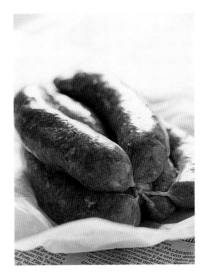

1 Remove the skin from the sausage, and make each into 3 balls.
2 Add the oil to a nonstick sauté pan (one that has a lid) and cook the sausage balls for 4 to 5 minutes, stirring occasionally, until they are brown all over. Remove from the pan and drain on paper towels.
3 Add the onion to the pan and sauté in the cooking juices for 5 minutes or until lightly browned.
4 Return the sausage balls to the pan, and stir in the orzo, tomatoes, broth, and oregano.
5 Cover and bring to simmering point, then cook for 10 minutes, stirring occasionally, until the orzo has absorbed much of the liquid and is nearly tender. Add more broth or water if all the liquid is used and the orzo needs more cooking.
6 When the orzo is tender, stir in the spinach, replace the lid, and cook for another 2 minutes or until the spinach has just wilted. Serve immediately.

**serving suggestions**
*Accompany with a crisp green salad.*

**storage**
*The stew is best served immediately, but can be kept in an airtight container in the refrigerator for 24 hours. Reheat until piping hot in a microwave oven. Not suitable for freezing.*

**allergens**
*Gluten (pasta, possibly sausages).*

# pot roasted chicken

This meal is a great one to do for visitors, because all the preparation is at the beginning and once it is in the oven, you can sit back and relax. If you prefer not to cook the asparagus at the end, simply add to the casserole about 30 minutes before you expect it to be ready.

serves  4 to 5
preparation time  15 minutes
cooking time  1½ hours

1 tablespoon vegetable oil
1 whole medium chicken
4 medium leeks (about 14 oz), trimmed and cut into
    2 inch lengths
12 oz new potatoes, scrubbed and halved, if large
1 large sweet potato (about 1 lb), peeled and cut
    into large cubes
3⅓ cups reduced sodium chicken broth
few parsley stems
2 bayleaves
14 oz asparagus, ½ inch cut off the stems

## VARIATION
*The chicken carcass can be boiled to make excellent broth for soups—just cover with water, add an onion, carrot, peppercorns, and a bay leaf or two, and simmer for 2-3 hours. Strain and chill or freeze.*

1 Preheat the oven to 400°F.
2 Fry the whole chicken in a large Dutch oven or casserole for 10 minutes, until lightly brown all over.
3 Place in a clean Dutch oven or ovenproof dish large enough to hold the chicken and the vegetables. Add the leeks, potatoes, and sweet potato.
4 Pour in the broth and add a few parsley stems. Cover and bake for one and a half hours, or until the chicken is cooked through and the juices run clear when tested with a sharp knife.
5 Lift out the chicken and place on a carving dish, cover with aluminum foil, and let rest for about 15 minutes. Meanwhile, keep the vegetables warm, and warm some serving dishes.
6 Lightly steam the asparagus using a basket steamer or purpose-made asparagus steamer.
7 When ready to serve, carve the chicken, remove the parsley stems, and accompany with the vegetables and gravy.

## storage
*The chicken can be removed from the bone and either frozen or kept refrigerated for 2 days. The vegetables can also be refrigerated for 2 days, but will be less rich in nutrients than when served freshly.*

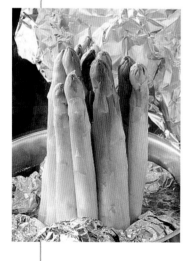

## STEAMING ASPARAGUS
*If you don't have a steamer, place your spears upright into a deep saucepan containing 4 inches simmering water, and wedge them into place using balls of aluminum foil. Cover with a dome of foil and simmer for 5 to 7 minutes, or until tender.*

# Italian chicken gnocchi

Gnocchi are little Italian dumplings, so they are ideal for cooking on top of a simple chicken stew. This comforting one-pot meal contains iron and folate, making it ideal in early pregnancy, when your needs for folic acid are especially high.

serves 2
preparation time 10 minutes
cooking time 20 minutes

*1 tablespoon olive oil*
*1 small onion, finely chopped*
*1 small fennel bulb, trimmed and coarsely chopped*
*5½ oz boneless chicken thighs, skinned and cubed*
*2 cloves garlic, crushed*
*1¾ cups tomato sauce*
*1 tablespoon chopped herbs, such as basil or oregano*
*5 cups small spinach leaves, washed*
*12 oz prepared gnocchi*

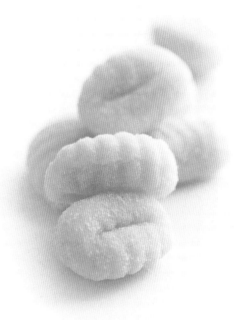

1 Heat the oil in a nonstick sauté pan and sauté the onion and fennel for 4 to 5 minutes to soften slightly.
2 Stir in the chicken and garlic and continue to sauté until the chicken is just starting to brown.
3 Pour in the tomato sauce and bring to simmering point. Then cover and heat gently for 10 minutes.
4 Meanwhile, put the spinach in a colander and pour boiling water over it to wilt it. Using a spatula, press down on the spinach to remove any excess water.
5 Stir the herbs and wilted spinach into the pan, and put the gnocchi on top. If the mixture looks a little dry, stir in a couple tablespoons of water.
6 Replace the lid and continue to cook for 3 to 4 minutes, until the gnocchi are hot through. Serve immediately.

**serving suggestions**
*You may want to sprinkle Parmesan cheese on top, or serve with a side salad.*

**storage**
*The cooked dish up to the end of step 3 can be refrigerated for up to 24 hours, or frozen. Simply reheat the chicken and sauce, and continue from step 4.*

**allergens**
*Gluten (wheat).*

one-pot dishes

# paella

Paella has to be a classic one-pot dish, and there are as many variations as there are cooks. Make this one to share with friends for a simple dinner, which has nutritional benefits for you and the baby, too. Using red bell peppers and fresh tomatoes alongside the peas provides plenty of vitamin C, and along with the zinc from the meat and fish, these nutrients will help to boost your immune system .

serves  4
preparation time  15 minutes
cooking time time  25 to 30 minutes

2 tablespoons olive oil
1 medium onion, finely chopped
9 oz boneless, skinless chicken breast or thigh,
    finely cubed
2 cloves garlic, crushed
2 large tomatoes,
1 large red bell pepper, sliced
½ teaspoon saffron threads, ground (optional)
1 teaspoon paprika
2 bay leaves
1⅓ cups paella or short grain rice
2 cups low-sodium chicken broth, hot
3½ oz shrimp of your choice, but if frozen, thawed
3½ oz squid, sliced
1 cup small peas

1 Heat the oil in a shallow skillet or paella pan, and
   sauté the onion for 5 minutes, or until lightly
   browned and soft.
2 Add the chicken and garlic, and cook over low heat
   for 5 minutes.
3 Meanwhile, skin (see page 123) and chop the
   tomatoes, removing the seeds, and slice the
   bell peppers.
4 Add these to the pan along with the saffron (if
   using), paprika, and bay leaves.
5 Stir in the rice and cook for a couple of minutes,
   stirring constantly to prevent it from sticking, before
   adding the broth. Stir through once and let the
   mixture simmer, uncovered, for about 15 minutes.

6 Finally add the shrimp, squid, and peas and cook for
   5 to 10 minutes, until cooked through. Stir in a little
   more broth or water, if needed.
7 If you are using raw shrimp, be sure they are pink
   throughout before serving. Check for seasoning,
   remove the bay leaves, and serve immediately.

### serving suggestions
*Accompany with  a crisp green salad.*

### allergens
*Fish and shellfish.*

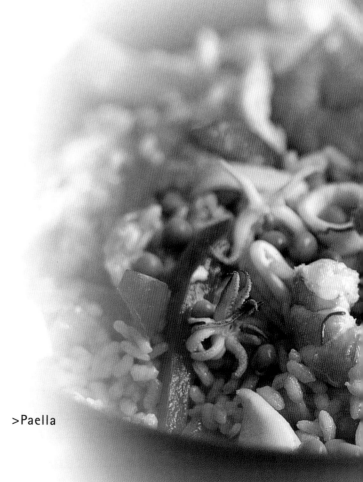

>Paella

# wild rice pilaf with fish, peas, and capers

In this easy-to-cook meal, the fish, which can be any white fish fillet of your choice, is gently steamed over the cooking rice and vegetables, keeping it moist and succulent. Fish is a pregnancy essential, and this recipe provides zinc and vitamins $B_3$ and $B_{12}$, as well as fiber.

serves 2
preparation time 5 minutes
cooking time 35 to 40 minutes

1 tablespoon vegetable oil
1 small leek or 4–5 scallions, finely sliced
¾ cup brown long grain rice and wild rice mix
1¼ cups water or fish broth
1 tablespoon capers
3 bay leaves
few strips lemon rind
¾ cup frozen peas, defrosted
9 oz skinless cod, halibut, or red snapper fillet
juice of ½ lemon

1 Heat the oil in a nonstick sauté pan (one that has a lid) and gently soften the leek or scallions for a few minutes without browning.
2 Wash the rice (see below), then stir it into the pan.
3 Pour in the water or broth, and add the capers, bay leaves, and lemon rind.
4 Stir well and bring to simmering point. Stir, cover, and cook gently for 20 to 25 minutes, or until the brown rice is starting to soften. Add a little more water or broth if there is none visible in the pan.
5 Stir in the peas and place the fish on top of the pilaf. Pour the lemon juice over the fish and replace the lid.
6 Cook for another 10 minutes, or until the fish becomes opaque and flakes easily. Serve immediately.

## serving suggestions
*Accompany with a few sliced ripe tomatoes.*

## allergens
*Fish.*

### WASHING RICE
*Most rice, but particularly basmati, benefits from having its excess starch removed by "washing." You can either place it in a strainer and run cold water over it or put it into a large bowl, cover with cold water, and stir with your fingers. When the rice settles, gently tip the bowl so the water drains away (it will be cloudy). Add more cold water and repeat as necessary untill the water runs clear.*

# casserole of duck and shallots with peaches

This dish is full of pregnancy essentials, namely zinc and copper, as well as being easy to prepare or cook in advance.

serves  2
preparation time  15 minutes
cooking time  2 hours

1 tablespoon vegetable oil
4 oz shallots or one medium onion, halved and sliced
2 large duck legs (about 1 lb, including bone)
2 peaches or nectarines, quartered and pitted
5 cardamon pods, coarsely crushed (optional) or a pinch of ground cloves
1 cup water
black pepper, to taste

## VARIATION
*Duck legs are available in supermarkets, however, if you can't find any, you can substitute them with chicken thighs, but reduce the cooking time by about half an hour.*

1 Preheat the oven to 350°F.
2 Wash the duck legs and pat dry with paper towels.
3 Heat the oil in a nonstick pan and gently sauté the shallots until lightly browned, stirring occasionally.
4 Add the duck, fruit, spice, and water, cover, and place in the oven for about 2 hours, or until the duck is really tender.
5 Season with black pepper and serve immediately.

### serving suggestions
*Eat with whole-grain rice and steamed broccoli or spinach.*

### storage
*The cooked dish can be kept in an airtight container and refrigerated for up to 2 days. Alternatively, it can be frozen for up to 3 months. Defrost overnight in a refrigerator before reheating until piping hot throughout.*

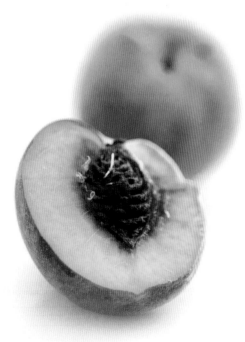

main dishes poultry

84

# chicken with pine nuts and prunes

Much derided but delicious and a great help to the digestive tract in pregnancy, prunes are a good source of iron as well as providing soluble fiber and potassium. This simple casserole with vitamin E-rich pine nuts is sweet and delicious, and can be frozen for use another time. The wine will, of course, be rendered nonalcoholic by the time you serve it, so is safe to add.

serves 4
preparation time  10 minutes
cooking time  40 to 45 minutes

*1 tablespoon vegetable oil*
*1 lb skinless, chicken thighs*
*1 medium onion, peeled, and sliced lengthwise*
*1½ cups pitted prunes*
*⅓ cup pine nuts*
*½ cup dry white wine*
*2 tablespoons chopped parsley*
*black pepper, to taste*

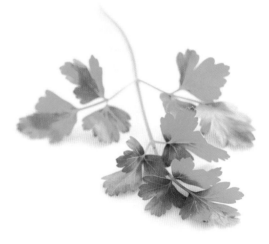

1 Heat the oil in a large, nonstick skillet (one that has a lid) and brown the chicken thighs over medium heat, turning the pieces occasionally.
2 Stir in the onion, lower the heat, and cover the pan. Continue to cook for 10 minutes.
3 Add the prunes, pine nuts, and wine and cook gently for another 10 to 15 minutes, or until the chicken is cooked through. Pierce the flesh with a sharp knife and look for clear, not pink, juices.
4 Stir in the parsley, check the seasoning, and serve immediately.

**serving suggestions**
*Eat with couscous, Almond Rice (page 136), and a green vegetable, such as snow peas, kale or spinach.*

**storage**
*The cooked dish may be kept in an airtight container and refrigerated for up to 2 days. Alternatively, it can be frozen for up to 2 months, defrosting in the refrigerator overnight and reheating until piping hot.*

**allergens**
*Pine nuts (not true nuts but some people are allergic to them).*

# chocolate and spicy chicken

If you are craving chocolate in pregnancy but want to stave off the urge to demolish a whole bar, try this Mexican-inspired recipe. You can make it in under half an hour—not as quick as unwrapping a chocolate bar, but it is much more nutritious.

serves 3
preparation time 5 minutes
cooking time 20 to 25 minutes

1 tablespoon olive oil
1 small red onion, finely chopped
10 oz skinless, boneless chicken thighs, each cut
    into 2 or 3 pieces
½ cup raisins
1 fresh red chile, finely chopped, optional
1 tablespoon cocoa powder
1 tablespoon cornstarch
pinch cinnamon
1 heaping tablespoon tomato paste
⅓ cup red wine

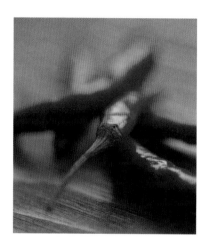

1 Heat the oil in a nonstick sauté pan (one that has a lid) and gently sauté the onion and chicken thighs, stirring often, for about 10 minutes, until browned all over.

2 You should have some cooking liquid remaining, but if not, add a tablespoon of water. Add the raisins, and chile (if using) and cover with the lid. Cook for another minute or two over low heat.

3 Meanwhile, mix the cocoa, cornstarch, cinammon, and tomato paste in a small bowl and gradually stir in the red wine and ½ cup water to make a sauce. Pour the sauce into the cooking liquid, and stir to coat everything.

4 Continue to cook for another few minutes, then check the chicken is cooked through. Test a piece by piercing the flesh with a sharp knife and looking to see if the juices run clear.

### serving suggestions
*Eat with a spoonful of yogurt or sour cream accompanied by Almond Rice, page 136 or soft corn or wheat tortillas or mashed sweet potato along with seasonal green vegetables.*

### storage
*This can be stored in an airtight container and refrigerated for up to 2 days. It can also be frozen for up to 3 months, and reheated until piping hot. If frozen, the sauce may separate a little on defrosting. If this happens, pour off the sauce and mix with a teaspoon of cornstarch. Then heat in a saucepan before mixing back in with the other ingredients and reheating the whole dish.*

### allergens
*Milk (yogurt).*

### CHILLI HEAT
*The volatile oil, capsaicin, while present in the whole pepper is concentrated in the seeds and pith. If you don't want your dish overly spicy, remove them with rubber glove covered fingers or use a small knife. If you don't wear rubber gloves, make sure you wash your hands afterwards.*

# duck and asian mushroom stir-fry

Duck breast fillets are available in supermarkets and make cooking a nutritious meal simple and quick. The combination of the duck and shitake mushrooms provides more than one quarter of your requirements for iron, with plenty of vitamins $B_{12}$ and C.

serves 2
preparation time 10 minutes
cooking time 10 minutes

1 tablespoon vegetable oil
8 oz duck breast fillets, cut into 1½ inch slices
5 oz shitake mushrooms, halved if large
2 scallions, cut into ½ inch pieces
½ yellow bell pepper, sliced
1 small red chile (optional), finely chopped
1 cup fresh bean sprouts
1 teaspoon grated ginger root
1 clove garlic crushed
4 teaspoons mirin rice wine or sweet sherry
4 teaspoons ketjap manis or light soy sauce

1 In a nonstick wok, heat the oil until hot and stir-fry the duck for 4 to 5 minutes, stirring all the time.
2 Add the mushrooms, onions, and bell pepper and cook for another minute or two
3 Add the chile, bean sprouts, garlic, and ginger, and stir-fry for two minutes.
4 Remove a piece of duck breast and cut in half to check it is cooked through; the juices should be clear and the meat pale brown, not pink.
5 If the duck is cooked, remove the wok from the heat and stir in the mirin and ketjap manis. If not, continue to cook a little longer before adding the wine and sauce.

## serving suggestions
*Divide the duck between 2 bowls and eat with plain noodles or coconut rice.*

## allergens
*Soy.*

# duck with cherries and leek mashed potatoes

This way of cooking duck breast is great for a special-occasion meal. Although duck is known for its fat content, it is not high in saturates, but the more healthy monounsaturated fat. If you want to cut the fat content, remove the skin after cooking and before eating.

serves 2
preparation time 25 minutes
cooking time 30 minutes

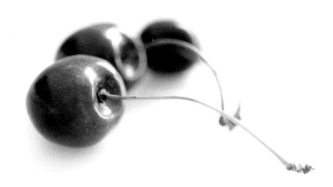

1 1/3 cups pitted fresh cherries
2/3 cup chicken broth
2½ tablespoons cherry preserves
1 tablespoon sherry or red wine vinegar
2 duck breast fillets (about 5 oz each)

**for the leek mashed potatoes**
1 tablespoon olive oil
1 medium leek, washed thoroughly and finely chopped
3 Yukon gold or russet potatoes, peeled
lowfat milk, to mash
black pepper

1 Simmer the cherries in the chicken broth for 10 to 15 minutes, until tender. Then stir the cherry preserves into the sauce along with the vinegar and heat until just simmering. Remove from heat and let cool a little.

2 Meanwhile, sauté the leeks in the olive oil over low heat for 10–15 minutes. Do not brown.

3 Boil the potatoes until tender.

4 Place the duck breasts, skin side down, in a skillet over medium–high heat and let brown. When the skin is crispy, turn over and cook the other side. Cook thoroughly until the juices run clear when the flesh is pierced by a sharp knife.

5 Drain and mash the potatoes with the milk, stir in the cooked leeks, and season with black pepper.

## serving suggestions
*Spoon the leek mashed potatoes onto warm plates and top with the duck breast. Serve with the cherry sauce and accompany with spinach, broccoli, or cauliflower.*

## storage
*The sauce and mashed potatoes can be frozen separately for up to 2 months, and reheated until piping hot. Alternatively, the sauce may be refrigerated for 48 hours.*

## allergens
*Milk.*

### PITTING CHERRIES
*A mechanical pitter makes it easy to remove the pits while retaining precious juices and the shape of the fruit.*

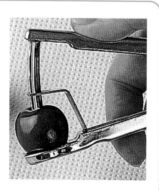

# mozzarella turkey with fig and ginger preserves

Thin turkey scallops or breast slices are quickly pan-fried or broiled and topped with a slice of mozzarella for added calcium and taste. When fresh figs are in season, this delicious preserves is a great partner for it or other turkey or chicken recipes. You'll have enough for four servings, so freeze some for when fresh figs are hard to come by.

serves  1
preparation time  10 minutes
cooking time  20 minutes

**for the preserves**
*1 tablespoon vegetable oil*
*1 small red onion, finely chopped*
*2 teaspoons grated ginger root*
*4 medium figs, washed, stem removed, and cut into
    8 pieces*
*⅓ cup water*
*2 teaspoons balsamic vinegar*

**for the turkey**
*2 turkey scallops or breast slices (about 3½ oz)*
*1½ oz slice of mozzarella*
*basil leaves, optional*

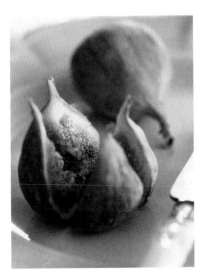

1 To make the preserves, heat the oil in a nonstick saucepan and sauté the onion gently until soft.
2 Stir in the ginger and figs and cook for a minute or two over medium heat before stirring in the water and vinegar.
3 Cover and let the ingredients simmer gently for 10 to 15 minutes, stirring occasionally until the mixture is thick and pulpy. Set aside while you prepare the turkey.
4 Preheat a broiler or ridged grill pan and lightly spray the turkey with oil.
5 Cook the turkey for 3 to 4 minutes on each side, until it is cooked through, then top with a couple of basil leaves, if using, and the mozzarella.
6 Put under the broiler for another couple of minutes, or until the cheese is softened.

**serving suggestions**
*Accompany with one quarter of the fig preserves and with new or mashed potatoes, and a seasonal green vegetable.*

**storage**
*The turkey is not suitable for storage, but the sauce may be kept in an airtight container and refrigerated for up to 2 days. Alternatively, the sauce may be frozen separately and should be piping hot when reheated.*

**allergens**
*Milk (mozzarella).*

main dishes poultry

# mushroom stuffed chicken with green lentils

Wonderfully rich in minerals, this stylish dish freezes well and looks impressive if you have people over. If you can't be bothered to make packages, you can add all the stuffing ingredients to the pan and omit the ham.

serves  4
preparation time  15 minutes
cooking time  1 to 1¼ hours

1 tablespoon olive oil
1 small onion, finely chopped
1½ cups finely chopped mushrooms
fine kitchen twine
4 pieces of prosciutto or Serrano ham
4 large, boned and skinned chicken thighs
4 large sprigs tarragon
black pepper
¾ cup green lentils
3 sticks celery chopped into ¾ inch lengths
1¾ cups diluted chicken broth
2 or 3 sprigs tarragon or 1 teaspoon dried

1 Preheat the oven to 350°F.
2 Heat the oil in a saucepan and gently sauté the onion and mushroom until soft. Let cool.
3 Cut 4 lengths of twine to about 16 inches each.
4 Place a slice of ham on a clean cutting board, then, on top of the ham and perpendicular to it, add a chicken thigh.
5 Spoon one quarter of the mushroom-and-onion mix onto the center of the thigh, then add a sprig of tarragon and a little black pepper.

6 Wrap the ham around the thigh and, with one length of twine, tie it in both directions.
7 Repeat until you have 4 chicken packages.
8 Put the lentils, celery, and remaining tarragon into a large ovenproof casserole and add the packages. Pour the broth over the chicken, cover the casserole, and place in the oven.
9 As they cook, the lentils will absorb much of the broth, so check occasionally that there is enough liquid, adding more water or broth as necessary.
10 Cook for a hour to an hour and a quarter, or until the chicken juices run clear when pierced with a sharp knife.
11 Remove the twine from the chicken packages and the sprigs of tarragon from the sauce before serving.

### serving suggestions
*Eat with kale, carrots, and brown rice, or* Gratin of Potato, *page 139.*

### storage
*The cooked dish can be refrigerated in an airtight container for 2 days. Alternatively, it can be frozen for up to 3 months, thawed overnight in the refrigerator, and reheated until piping hot.*

### allergens
*Celery.*

# sesame and coriander chicken with mango salsa

Chicken thighs are a better source of minerals, such as zinc and iron, than breasts. Vitamin C, of course, helps your body absorb iron and along with energy releasing niacin, and essential vitamin $B_{12}$, this dish provides a gestational nutritional boost. And it also tastes great, too.

serves 2
preparation time 15 minutes
cooking time 15 minutes

*4 small or 2 large boned, skinless chicken thighs*
*1 tablespoon olive oil*
*1 tablespoon sesame seeds*
*1 tablespoon coriander seeds, lightly crushed*
*juice of ½ lime*
*2 cloves garlic, crushed*

### mango salsa
*½ large mango or ½ cup mango cubes*
*juice of ½ small lemon or lime*
*½ small red onion*
*½ red bell pepper*
*1 teaspoon chopped cilantro*
*1 small chile (optional), very finely chopped*

1 Trim any visible fat from the chicken thighs.
2 Mix together the next 5 ingredients in a bowl large enough to hold the chicken pieces. Add the chicken and stir to coat with the marinade. Cover and refrigerate while you prepare the salsa.
3 Cut the mango into ½ inch cubes and place in a serving bowl. Pour the lemon or lime juice over the cubes.
4 Finely slice the red onion and cut the bell pepper into small pieces or slices, then add both to the bowl of mango.
5 Stir in the cilantro and chile, if using, and chill until required.

6 Heat a ridged grill pan or broiler pan and remove the chicken from the refrigerator.
7 Place the thighs on the hot grill or broiler pan. Cook for 5 minutes on each side, then test for doneness. Insert a knife into the flesh and check to see the juices run clear. If not, cook for a couple minutes longer.

### serving suggestions
*Accompany with the salsa and some boiled new potatoes or coconut rice.*

### storage
*The chicken thighs can be eaten cold so can be refrigerated for up to 48 hours. The salsa is best within 24 hours. Neither is suitable for freezing.*

### allergens
*Sesame.*

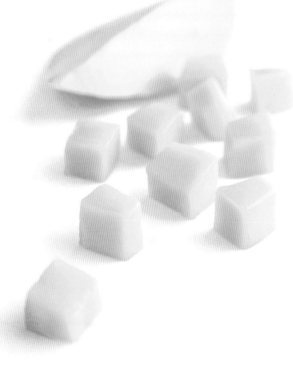

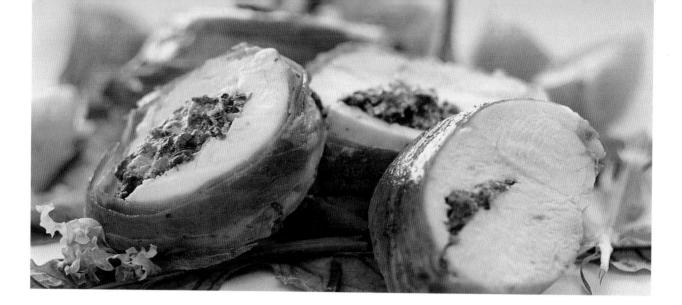

# spinach stuffed chicken breasts with prosciutto

A simple and elegant dish that is wonderful to serve for a dinner party or a special dinner for two. The spinach filling provides essential vitamin A.

serves  2
preparation time  15 minutes
cooking time  35 minutes

2 boneless chicken breasts, skinned
1¾ cups thawed, chopped frozen spinach, drained
1 rounded tablespoon reduced-fat mascarpone cheese
1 tablespoon parsley, chopped
zest of ½ lemon, grated
pinch of grated nutmeg
2 large or 4 small slices prosciutto
toothpicks or kitchen twine
1 teaspoon olive oil

1 Preheat the oven to 350°F.
2 Slice horizontally into each chicken breast to make a pocket.
3 Mix the drained spinach with the mascarpone, parsley, lemon, and nutmeg.
4 Spoon half the filling into each pocket.

5 Lay the prosciutto on a piece of wax paper and place the stuffed breast on top. Wrap the prosciutto around the chicken, using the paper to help position it. Secure with toothpicks or twine.
6 Heat the oil in a nonstick skillet and cook the breasts on each side for about 3 minutes, or until just browned.
7 Transfer to an ovenproof dish, cover, and bake for about 30 minutes, or until the juices of the flesh run clear when pierced with a knife.
8 Remove the toothpicks or twine and slice, if desired.

## serving suggestions
*Eat with boiled new potatoes or mashed sweet potatoes and seasonal greens.*

## allergens
*Milk (mascarpone).*

# STUFF IT!

Chicken and turkey are extremely versatile, and there are many different recipes you can make with a few simple ingredients. Instead of simply frying or broiling a chicken or turkey cutlet or scallop, it's easy to bake the chicken or turkey with a filling that adds nutrients to your diet, and that looks and tastes great, too. Meat from flocks that are allowed to roam can have a more flavorsome taste, so try to buy locally produced poultry from a reliable source.

## QUANTITIES
These fillings make enough to stuff two chicken or two turkey cutlets or scallops.

## mushroom and onion
Sauté one coarsely chopped small onion with 4 to 5 chopped cremini mushrooms in 1 teaspoon of olive oil. Mix in the grated zest of half a lemon and some black pepper.

## sun-dried tomato and cheese
Drain 4 pieces of sun-dried tomatoes in oil on some paper towels and coarsely chop. Stir into 3 tablespoons reduced-fat cream cheese along with one clove of crushed garlic and a little black pepper.

## marinated artichoke and tarragon
Drain 2 marinated artichokes on some paper towels, then coarsely chop. Mix with the zest of one orange and a few sprigs of fresh tarragon.

## walnut, prune, and cinnamon
Chop 6 pitted prunes with ¼ cup walnut pieces and stir in a pinch of ground cinnamon.

> ### VARIATION
> *For alternative recipes, see* Spinach Stuffed Chicken Breasts with Prosciutto and Mushroom, *page 92, and* Mushroom Stuffed Chicken with Green Lentils, *page 90.*

## HOW TO STUFF AND WRAP A CHICKEN OR TURKEY CUTLET OR SCALLOP

1 Once you have made the filling, you will need to make a large enough pocket in the meat to hold your filling, using a sharp knife. Then add the filling to the pocket. Decide if you want to first wrap the chicken or turkey in bacon, prosciutto, or ham (Serrano ham works well) to add moistness to the poultry, or just secure the filling with either toothpicks or kitchen twine.

2 If you are using bacon or ham to wrap, flatten the slice out on a piece of wax paper or lightly oiled aluminum foil and lay the stuffed chicken or turkey on top. Then wrap the cutlet or scallop up with it, using the paper or foil to help you. Secure with toothpicks or kitchen twine.

3 Transfer the package, still in the foil or wax paper, to a roasting pan or baking sheet and cook in a preheated oven at 375°F for 30 minutes. Then open the foil or peel off the paper and let the chicken or turkey brown for 10 minutes or until the juices in the poultry run clear when pierced with a knife.

4 Serve, remembering to remove the toothpicks or twine.

# turkey herb burgers with fruity salsa

Ground turkey is low in fat, and high in vitamin $B_3$, or niacin, which helps release energy. Combined with some herbs and served with a roll, fruity salsa, and mustardy watercress, you'll be providing great nutrition for your baby as well as having a tasty meal. If you buy a 1 pound package of meat, you can use half for this recipe and freeze the rest to use later, or double up on the ingredients and make and freeze the whole batch.

serves  2 to 3
preparation time  15 minutes
cooking time  20 to 25 minutes

*8 oz ground turkey*
*½ small onion, coarsely chopped*
*2 cloves of garlic*
*2 or 3 stems fresh parsley, or ½ teaspoon dried*
*flour*
*1 tablespoon vegetable oil*

### for the fruity salsa
*1 large ripe nectarine or peach, skin and pit removed*
*1 ripe medium tomato, skinned*
*juice of one medium orange or ¼ cup unsweetened juice*
*1 teaspoon packed dark brown sugar, optional*

### to serve
*2 to 3 whole wheat or multi-seed rolls*
*olive spread*
*handful of watercress*

1 Place the ground turkey, onion, garlic, and parsley into a processor and pulse until just combined.
2 Remove and, using a little flour on your hands to prevent the meat from sticking, shape into 2 to 3 patties, depending on appetite. Chill.
3 Meanwhile, coarsely chop the peach or nectarine and tomato and put into a small saucepan.
4 Stir in the orange juice and cook gently for about 10 to 15 minutes, until the fruit is tender, adding more juice if the salsa looks dry.
5 Taste, and add a little sugar, if required. Let cool.
6 Heat the oil oil in a skillet and gently cook the patties for 5 to 6 minutes each side, until the juices run clear when pierced with a knife. Alternatively, brush lightly with oil and broil.
7 Warm the rolls and lightly spread with olive spread. Top with the burgers and watercress and serve with the salsa.

### storage
*Once cooked, the turkey burgers are not suitable for reheating, but while raw they can be wrapped individually in plastic wrap and frozen for up to one month. Defrost in the refrigerator and cook as above. The sauce can be stored in the refrigerator for 2 to 3 days, although it will lose B vitamins and vitamin C when stored and reheated.*

### allergens
*Wheat (gluten).*

### VARIATION
*You can make the salsa using canned peaches in juice. Just reduce the amount of orange juice you use. Other variations would be to add vitamin A rich mango, or some pitted dried apricots or a few raisins, and some allspice or ground cloves.*

# teriyaki turkey with sesame cucumber salad

This Japanese-style dish is high on flavor and low in saturated fat. It makes a great light lunch or you can add some rice to turn it into a more substantial evening meal. Turkey is an unusually good source of niacin (vitamin $B_3$). Both the marinade and salad dressing contain ginger root, which can be a great help in preventing pregnancy nausea.

serves  2
preparation time   15 minutes
cooking time   10 minutes

### for the teriyaki marinade
2 tablespoons mirin rice wine or sweet sherry
4 teaspoons soy sauce, preferably reduced sodium
1 teaspoon grated lime zest
2 teaspoons grated ginger root
juice of ½ lime

4 small turkey scallops (about 2 oz each)
  or 2 larger turkey cutlets

### for the sesame cucumber salad
½ cucumber
2 cloves garlic, crushed
2 teaspoons grated ginger root
2 tablespoons canola or sunflower oil
pinch of sugar
1 to 2 tablespoons chopped fresh cilantro
1 heaping tablespoon sesame seeds, toasted

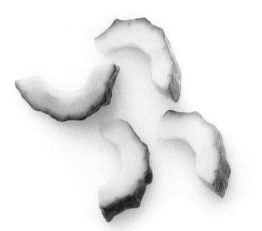

1 Mix together all the marinade ingredients in a bowl and stir in the turkey scallops so they are coated with the marinade. Cover and refrigerate.
2 Cut the cucumber in half lengthwise and remove the seeds so the cucumber pieces are hollowed out. Cut the lengths into fat slices, each of which will resemble a semicircle.
3 Mix together the garlic, ginger, oil, and sugar to make a thick dressing and stir in the cucumber pieces.
4 Add the cilantro and sesame seeds and chill while you cook the turkey.
5 Preheat a ridged grill pan or broiler pan. Remove the turkey from the marinade and wipe off any excess; it should just have a little clinging to it.
6 Grill or broil the turkey on one side for 3 to 4 minutes, then turn to cook the other side a similar time. Depending on the thickness of the turkey, you may need to cook for another minute or so until the flesh is cooked through and the juices run clear.

### serving suggestions
*Eat with the salad and add rice or udon noodles for a more substantial meal.*

### storage
*The salad is best eaten within 24 hours. The cooked turkey is not suitable for reheating but you could eat any remaining cold within 24 hours with a different salad or sliced in a wrap or tortilla.*

### allergens
*Sesame, soy.*

> ## COOK'S TIP
> *Choose reduced-sodium soy sauce can help to keep your sodium intake down.*

# pork with pineapple

This recipe provides huge amounts of energy-releasing B vitamins, even when nutrient losses due to cooking are accounted for. You can try broiling or grilling the fresh pineapple on a barbecue for a different take on this classic combination.

serves  2
preparation time  15 minutes
cooking time  15 minutes

10½ oz pork tenderloin, cut into ¾ inch wide slices
1 cup pineapple juice, ideally fresh
1 clove garlic, crushed (optional)
1 tablespoon vegetable oil
1 medium onion, finely chopped
1 large stick celery, washed and sliced
1 medium carrot, peeled and sliced
4 thinly sliced disks of pineapple

1 Put the pork slices and pineapple juice into a bowl with the garlic, if using. Let stand for 10 minutes.
2 Meanwhile, heat the oil in a nonstick saucepan and add the onion, celery, and carrot. Cover and cook over low heat for 5 minutes, until soft but not browned.
3 Drain the pork, saving the juice. Pat the pork dry on some paper towels.
4 Add the pineapple juice to the vegetable mixture and simmer until the vegetables are just tender, adding a little water if the mixture is too dry.
5 Heat a ridged grill pan and spray with cooking oil. When hot, cook the pineapple slices briefly for 2 to 3 minutes to achieve a grilled appearance. Put to one side.
6 Respray the pan and cook the sliced pork for a few minutes on each side until the juices run clear.
7 Serve the pork with the pineapple and the vegetable sauce poured over top.

serving suggestions
*Eat with cooked pearl barley or brown rice, and a seasonal green vegetable.*

storage
*The sauce may be refrigerated or frozen but the pork is best freshly cooked.*

allergens
*Celery.*

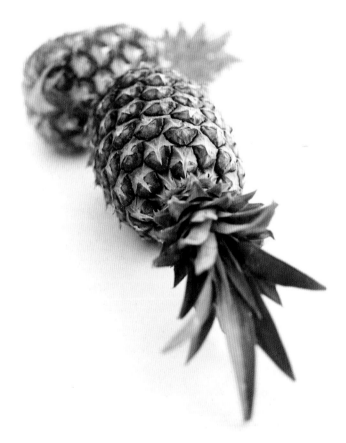

> **FOOD SAFETY**
> *Be sure the pork is properly cooked, checking that the juices run clear when you insert a sharp knife.*

# Chinese pork with plums

Pork is a good source of thiamin (vitamin $B_1$), which helps release energy from foods, so it is essential for your baby's overall growth and development as well as keeping you well.

serves 2
preparation time 15 minutes
cooking time 15 minutes

1 tablespoon vegetable oil
1 (9–10 oz) pork tenderloin, cut into ½ inch slices
1 medium red onion, finely sliced
3 cloves garlic, chopped
1¼ inch piece fresh ginger, peeled and cut into fine matchsticks
1 teaspoon Chinese five-spice powder
8 smallish plums, pitted and quartered
1 tablespoon packed light brown sugar
½ cup water

1 Heat the oven to 300°F.
2 Heat 1 teaspoon of the oil in a nonstick skillet, the pork, and cook for 5 minutes or until lightly browned, then turn and cook for another few minutes until the juices run clear. Keep warm in a covered dish in the oven.
3 Heat the remaining oil in the pan and sauté the onion and garlic for a minute or two.
4 Add the ginger, five-spice powder, plums, sugar, and water and let simmer gently for 10 minutes, or until the plums are softened.
5 Pour the plum sauce over the pork and serve.

**serving suggestions**
*Eat with boiled noodles and stir-fried bok choy or other green vegetable.*

**storage**
*The sauce may be refrigerated or frozen but the pork is best freshly cooked.*

**allergens**
*Milk (if using yogurt or cream).*

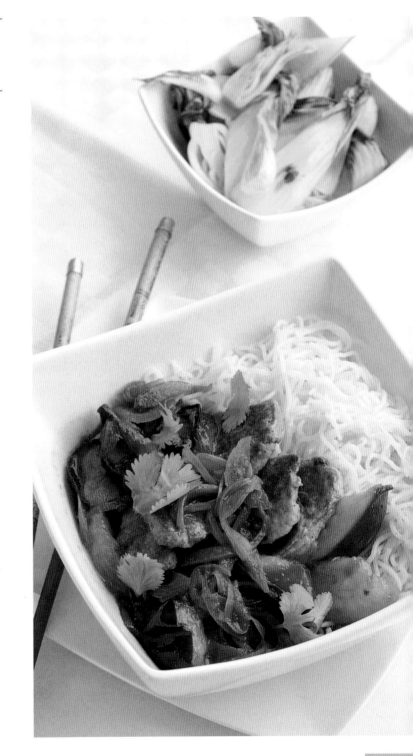

# Hungarian goulash

Made with smoked paprika and red instead of green bell peppers, this dish is both high in zinc and vitamin A. It freezes well, so it is a great one to make for later in pregnancy, or for when your baby has arrived and you may have little time or energy to cook.

serves 4
preparation time 10 minutes
cooking time 1 hour 45 minutes to 2 hours

1 tablespoon vegetable oil
1 medium onion, halved and then sliced
3 cloves garlic, crushed
1 tablespoon all-purpose flour or cornstarch
1 tablespoon smoked paprika
1 lb lean, boneless chuck shoulder steak, cut into
  ¾ inch cubes
1 cup beef broth
1 (14½ oz) can diced tomatoes
2 medium red bell peppers, cut into large pieces

1 Preheat the oven to 325°F.
2 Heat the oil in a large ovenproof casserole o rDutch oven and sauté the onion for 5 minutes, or until lightly browned. Stir in the garlic and sauté for another minute or so.
3 Meanwhile place the flour and paprika in a clean plastic food bag and drop in the meat. Shake to coat with the flour.
4 Transfer the floured meat and any remaining seasoned flour into the casserole and stir briefly.
5 Add the broth, tomatoes, and red bell peppers and bring slowly to simmering point, stirring often.
6 Cover and transfer the casserole to the oven and cook for 1½ hours. Stir, and return to the oven for 15 to 30 minutes, until the meat is really tender.

### serving suggestions
Eat with *Gratin of Potato*, page 139 and a green vegetable.

### storage
*The goulash may be kept in an airtight container and refrigerated for up to 2 days, or frozen for up to 3 months. Defrost overnight in the refrigerator and ideally reheat in a microwave oven until piping hot.*

### allergens
*Wheat (gluten) if wheat flour used.*

### VARIATION
*If you like your goulash hot, choose hot smoked paprika or add 1 teaspoon chili powder to the flour mixture. You may want to serve sour cream or yogurt with a spicier goulash.*

# beef in beer

Reputed as helpful for promoting breast-milk production, stout helps tenderize the beef in this winter-warming casserole. Adding a few carrots provides your baby with plenty of vitamin A for her eye development as well as for boosting your immune system. Freeze extra portions for when your baby has arrived.

serves  4
preparation time  10 minutes
cooking time  1½ to 2 hours

2 tablespoons vegetable oil
2 medium onions, sliced
1 rounded tablespoon all-purpose flour or
    cornstarch
black pepper, to taste
1 teaspoon dried thyme or few fresh thyme sprigs
1 lb lean, boneless chuck shoulder steak, cut into
    1 inch pieces
5 carrots, cut into chunks
1½ cups stout or dark ale
1 tablespoon Worcestershire sauce or mushroom
    ketchup
3 cups sliced open cap mushrooms

1 Preheat the oven to 325°F.
2 Heat the oil in a skillet and sauté the onions for about
    5 minutes, until just softening.
3 Meanwhile, place the flour in a clean plastic food bag
    and season with the black pepper and thyme.
4 Drop in the pieces of steak and shake to coat with the
    seasoned flour.
5 Transfer the onions to an ovenproof casserole dish, and
    add the meat, any remaining flour, and the carrots.
6 Pour the stout over the meat and stir in the
    Worcestershire sauce.
7 Cover and bake in the oven for 1 hour.
8 Remove the casserole from the oven and stir in the
    mushrooms. Continue to cook for 30 to 60 minutes,
    until the beef is tender.

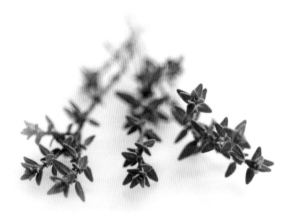

### serving suggestions
*Eat with baked potatoes that have cooked alongside the stew, and boiled or stir-fried cabbage or kale.*

### storage
*The stew can be refrigerated for 2 days or frozen for up to 2 months. Defrost overnight in the refrigerator and reheat until piping hot.*

### allergens
*Fish (if using Worcestershire sauce), gluten (if wheat flour used). Use cornstarch if sensitive to wheat.*

## COOK'S TIP
*Using a good quality, thick nonstick sauté pan with a lid is a great way to reduce the amount of fat you use in cooking.*

# baked beef and sour cherries

Beef is a marvelous source of the B vitamins and minerals and one portion of this recipe boasts more than a day's supply of vitamins $B_3$ and $B_{12}$, as well as zinc and iron. It contains sweetened sour cherries, which add a piquancy to the taste and vitamin A for your baby. The recipe uses red wine, but you don't need worry; it will just impart flavor, not alcohol, because the alcohol will burn off. Make a batch to enjoy now or freeze for when your baby has arrived and time is short.

serves  4

preparation time  10 minutes

cooking time  2 to 2½ hours

1 rounded tablespoon all-purpose flour or
  cornstarch
1 teaspoon mixed dried herbs, or 1 bouquet garni
1 lb lean, boneless shoulder chuck steak, cut into
  ¾ inch cubes
1 tablespoon canola oil
1 large onion, coarsely chopped
4 cloves garlic, crushed
1 cup dried sour sweetened cherries
1 cup red wine (or replace with water)
½ cup water
black pepper and salt, if required

1 Preheat the oven to 325°F.
2 Place the flour and mixed herbs in a clean plastic
  food bag and add the meat. Shake the bag to coat
  the meat with the flour and herbs.
3 Heat the oil in a nonstick saucepan. Gently brown
  the onions and garlic before transferring them to a
  large casserole or ovenproof dish that has a lid.
4 Add the meat and cherries and stir in the wine
  and water.
5 Cover the casserole or dish and place in the oven
  for 2 hours, then remove and stir. If the meat is
  already tender, it is ready to serve; if it needs longer,
  return the casserole or dish to the oven for another
  20 to 30 minutes.
6 Check the seasoning and serve.

### serving suggestions
*Eat with whole-grain rice and steamed broccoli or spinach.*

### storage
*You can freeze this in an airtight container for 2 to 3 months, or keep in the refrigerator for 48 hours. Defrost in the refrigerator overnight and reheat until piping hot.*

### allergens
*Wheat (gluten) if wheat flour used. Use cornstarch if sensitive to wheat.*

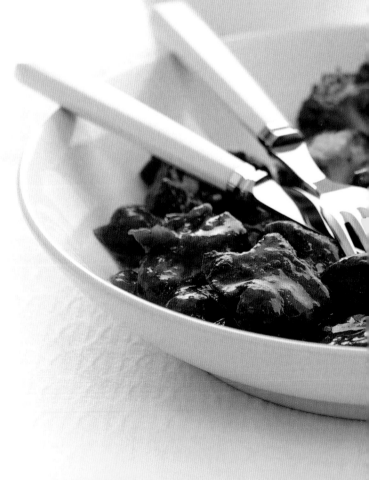

>baked beef and sour cherries

# steak and broccoli with noodles

No meal is much faster than a stir-fry, and it is worth treating yourself to a small piece of steak to make this quick and iron-rich dish. If available, try some different mushrooms for a change, using Japanese enoki or buna shimeji for added flavor.

serves 2
preparation time 10 minutes
cooking time 5 to 10 minutes

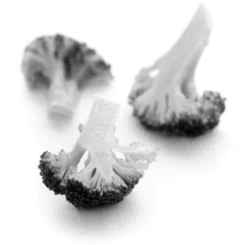

4 or 5 florets broccoli, cut into smaller florets
2 nests or about 4 oz dry noodles
2 tablespoons vegetable oil
8 oz lean sirloin or tenderloin steak, cut into
  bite-size chunks
1 red onion, finely sliced
2 or 3 cloves garlic, crushed
5 oz mushrooms (enoki, buna shimeji or button),
  finely sliced
2 tablespoons oyster sauce

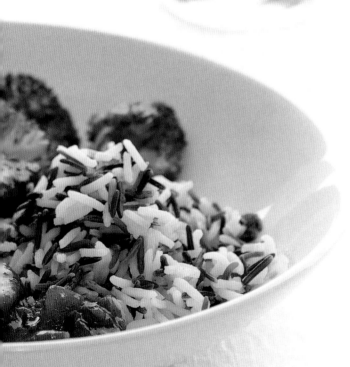

1 Steam the broccoli florets for 2 to 3 minutes to blanch them, then put to one side while you cook the noodles according to the package directions.
2 Meanwhile, heat the oil in a nonstick wok or large skillet and cook the steak for 2 to 3 minutes, then add the onion and garlic.
3 Stir-fry the beef, onion, and garlic for a minute or two longer, then add the mushrooms and blanched broccoli. Continue to cook for a minute or so, or until the mushrooms have just softened.
4 Drain the noodles and stir into the beef mixture along with the oyster sauce.
5 Serve immediately in warm dishes.

## allergens
*Wheat (noodles), soy, and shellfish (check the oyster sauce label).*

# BROIL OR GRILL IT ...

There are many cuts of meat or poultry that are quickly cooked by putting them under the broiler, on a barbeque grill rack, on a stove-top ridged grill pan, or simply pan-frying. Here, you will find some basic information on how to cook a variety of cuts, as well as a host of different marinades, hot and cold sauces, and salsas you can serve them with.

## the basics

Any meat or poultry that is to be cooked quickly by, say, broiling needs to be tender, and a little fat, whether present in the flesh, or lightly brushed on the surface keeps the meat moist. Grilling using a ridged cast iron pan allows any fat to drain off the meat, and provides characteristic stripes.

## best cuts to use

**Beef** steaks—tenderloin or sirloin

**Lamb** loin or leg chops or cutlets, noisettes (boned, rolled loin chop)

**Pork** leg cutlets or scallops, loin chops, tenderloin, spareribs

**Venison** haunch, loin, or shoulder "steaks" from young animals or if supermarket package recommends broiling

**Chicken** thigh, drumstick, breast, wing—with skin on—can remove before serving

**Turkey** breast as cutlet or scallop—if very lean, brush with oil or marinade first

**Ostrich** thigh steaks or back tenderloin medallions

**Duck** breast cooked with pierced skin, broiled skin side up, or grilled skin side down

## broiling

1 Preheat the broiler.
2 Check the thickness of the meat. Put thinner cuts closer to the heat source and thicker cuts farther away, so you don't burn the meat before the middle is cooked.
3 Turn and brush the meat/poultry with a little oil or marinade every few minutes during broiling to keep it moist.

## grilling

1 Preheat the ridged grill pan.
2 Brush the meat with oil and place on the hot grill pan. (If the grill pan is really hot when you start, you may not need to brush the meat with oil, but this may also depend on the fat content of what you are cooking.)
3 Leave the meat/poultry for a few minutes without turning to allow searing, then using tongs turn over.
3 If the meat is thick, you may need to turn over again.
4 The timings are similar to broiling but may be a little less for thinner cuts.
5 Cuts more than 1¼ inches thick are not suitable for grilling.

## pan-frying

Broiling and grilling use less fat than pan-frying, so are a healthier cooking method.
1 Put 1 to 2 tablespoons of vegetable oil into a nonstick pan and heat until the oil is hot but not smoking.

| Broiling times | | | |
|---|---|---|---|
| Cut | Rare* | Medium | Well done |
| Beef, steaks (not tenderloin) | 5-6 mins | 8-12 mins | 15-18 mins |
| tenderloin steak | 3-5 mins | 6-7 mins | 8-10 mins |
| Pork chops or cutlets | | 10-14 mins | |
| Lamb chops or cutlets | | 10-14 mins | |
| Chicken breast | | | 15-20 mins |
| Turkey cutlet | | | 12-15 mins |
| Duck breast | | | 15-20 mins |

* in pregnancy you should not eat any meat that is rare or undercooked.

2 Add the meat/poultry and cook for 2 to 3 minutes without turning to let the surface seal.
3 Let cook well on one side before turning with tongs to cook on the reverse.
4 Drain the food on paper towels before serving.

## marinades

Marinades are a popular way of adding flavor to a fairly bland cut. If you want to make your own, you'll need something to provide acid and an oil to carry flavor. Then you can try an endless range of herbs and spices. Whatever you marinate must go in the refrigerator to minimize the risk of food poisoning.

Juices, vinegars, and wines are acidic and will break down the protein in the meat, which may not so much tenderize as to make the surface of the meat mushy. So to make sure you don't overdo the timing, look at the timing suggestions below,

### herb marinade

*2/3 cup wine (red for beef or lamb; white for pork)*
*1/4 cup oil (canalo has a neutral flavor, but you can use olive oil)*
*1/4 cup wine vinegar*
*2 or 3 cloves garlic, crushed*
*2 bay leaves*
*1 tablespoon chopped fresh herbs of your choosing e.g parsley, sage, tarragon, rosemary*

1 Place all the ingredients in a screw-top jar or sealable container and shake well.
2 Pour the marinade over the meat and stir well.
3 Cover and refrigerate for a minimum of 1 hour, turning occasionally.
4 Remove the meat from the marinade and drain on paper towels.

### chicken marinade

Chicken is tender so doesn't need that much tenderizing, but a marinade that adds flavor before cooking is great.

*2 or 3 tablespoons olive oil*
*grated zest of one lime or 1/2 lemon*
*black pepper*
*1 clove garlic, crushed*
*any of the following:*
  *1 tablespoon grainy mustard; 1 teaspoon dried herbs or 1 tablespoon fresh; 2 teaspoon grated ginger root; 2 teaspoon grated lemongrass; 1 teaspoon dried red pepper flakes.*

1 Mix all the ingredients in the container to be used for marinating.
2 Add the chicken pieces and stir well.
3 Cover and refrigerate for 15 to 30 minutes
4 Remove and cook, wiping off any excess marinade, if required.

## some great combos

- Grilled venison steak with *Wild Mushroom and Rosemary Sauce*
- Grilled lamb chop with *Blackberry Sauce*
- Grilled pork loin chop with *Apple, Sage, and Walnut Sauce*
- Barbequed lamb leg cutlets with *Kachumbari*
- Pan-fried turkey scallops with *Mango Salsa*
- Grilled sirloin steak with *Fruity Sauce*
- Broiled Chicken drumsticks with *Peanut Satay Sauce*
- Pan-fried chicken breasts with *Tarragon Sauce*
- *Lamb and Bell Pepper Koftas with Tzatziki*

### Maximum marinade times

| Chicken | Pork | Lamb | Beef |
|---------|------|------|------|
| 2 hours | 4 hours | 8 hours | 24 hours |

**COOK'S TIP**
*Making a cut in the surface of the meat will allow the marinade to penetrate.*

# sauces

Sauces provide moisture for broiled or grilled meat as well as add contrasting or enhancing flavors. They can also be a way of adding vitamins and minerals to your meal, although the quantity consumed is not usually enough to provide a significant boost. The following recipes—both warm and cold sauces—are ideal accompaniments to many different types of meats and poultry.

## apple, sage, and walnut sauce

Pork chops particularly cry out for applesauce, and this one provides sage for a punch and walnuts for additional texture, healthy oils, and vitamin E.

serves 4
preparation time 5 minutes
cooking time 10 to 15 minutes

*1 medium cooking apple, such as Granny Smith, peeled and cubed*
*½ cup unsweetened apple cider*
*3-4 large sage leaves, finely chopped or 1 teaspoon dried rubbed sage*
*⅓ cup finely chopped walnuts*

1 Put the apple, juic,e and sage into a nonstick saucepan and cook over gentle heat until the apple is tender and breaks up. Add a little more juice, if required.
2 Add the walnuts, check the seasoning, adding more sage and black pepper, if required.
3 Either cool to use later or serve with broiled meat, such as pork, immediately.

### serving suggestions
*Use to accompany any broiled or grilled pork or other meat.*

## blackberry sauce

An easy, delicious sauce to accompany broiled or grilled meat. This sauce, which can be frozen, tastes especially good with venison, but would make an ideal accompaniment to duck or a piece of steak. Don't worry about the wine—any alcohol will be boiled off.

serves 4
preparation time 5 minutes
cooking time 15 minutes

*½ cup red wine*
*1½ cups blackberries*
*2 cardamom pods, crushed (optional)*
*3 tablespoons red currant, blueberry, or grape jelly*

1 Put the wine, blackberries, and cardamom into a saucepan and bring to a boil.
2 Boil gently for about 10 minutes, or until the mixture is halved in volume.
3 Stir in the jelly, and let simmer for a minute or two.
4 Either cool to use later or serve with broiled meat immediately.

### serving suggestions
*Use to accompany venison, steak, or duck.*

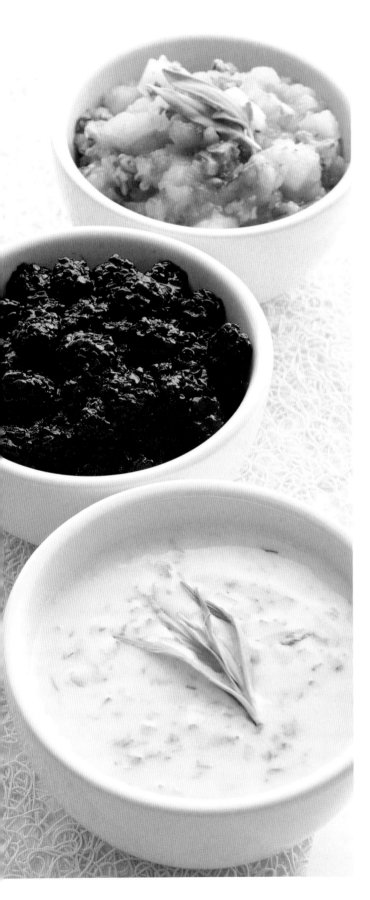

## tarragon sauce

An anise-scented sauce is a classic accompaniment to chicken, but this version is lower in fat than the classic recipe. By using a little cornstarch to stabilize the sauce, you can swap heavy cream for reduced-fat crème fraiche or sour cream.

serves 4
preparation time 5 minutes
cooking time 15 minutes

1 tablespoon vegetable oil
1 small onion or medium shallot, minced
1 cup lowsodium chicken broth
1 tablespoon fresh chopped tarragon
1 teaspoon cornstarch
¼ cup reduced-fat crème fraiche

1 Heat the oil in a saucepan and sauté the onion until just starting to brown.
2 Add the chicken broth, bring to a boil, and let boil gently for 10 or so minutes, or until the mixture is halved in volume.
3 Stir in the tarragon and let simmer for a minute or two.
4 Mix the cornstarch with a tablespoon of water and stir it into the broth, then bring to simmering point.
5 Stir in the crème fraiche over low heat. Either cool to use later or serve with broiled meat immediately.

### serving suggestions
*Serve with chicken or turkey cutlets or scallops.*

### STORAGE
*The sauces on these two pages may be kept in an airtight container and refrigerated for up to 2 days. Alternatively, the sauce smay be frozen separately but when reheating, they must reach a boil before serving.*

## peanut satay sauce

Now peanuts are back on the menu for moms-to-be—unless, of course, you are allergic to them—you can enjoy their creaminess in simple sauces such as this. It is a good companion for marinated kebabs, lamb, chicken, or even shrimp, and adds small quantities of some key minerals, such as iron, zinc, and copper.

- - - - - - - - - - - - - - - - - - - - - - - - - - - - - - - - - -
serves  4
preparation time  5 minutes
cooking time  5 minutes
- - - - - - - - - - - - - - - - - - - - - - - - - - - - - - - - - -

2 scallions, chopped into fine slices
1 small red chile, finely chopped (optional)
⅓ cup chunky peanut butter
4 teaspoons unsweetened coconut cream
  (if you can't find cream, scoop it from
  the top of a can of coconut milk)
1 teaspoon soy sauce
1 teaspoon Thai fish sauce
¾ cup water
juice of 1 lime

1 Put all the ingredients except the lime into a saucepan and, stirring all the time, bring to simmering point.
2 Remove from the heat and stir in the lime juice.
3 Serve hot.

### serving suggestions
*Serve with chicken or lamb kabobs.*

### storage
*The sauce may be kept in an airtight container and refrigerated for 2 days.*

### allergens
*Peanuts, soy.*

## wild mushroom and rosemary sauce

You can you can buy many different types of wild mushrooms—from chanterelle to shitake or porcini. Each variety has different amount of the B vitamins and iron, but not usually enough in a sauce to get excited about.

- - - - - - - - - - - - - - - - - - - - - - - - - - - - - - - - - -
serves  4
preparation time  5 minutes
cooking time  15 minutes
- - - - - - - - - - - - - - - - - - - - - - - - - - - - - - - - - -

2 tablespoons spread high in monounsaturates, such as olive spread
7 oz mixed mushrooms, such as 5 oz cremini and 2 oz wild; sliced or if small, left whole
1 tablespoon all-purpose flour
1 cup low-sodium beef broth
1 tablespoon fresh chopped rosemary

1 Heat the spread in a nonstick saucepan and sauté the mushrooms for 5 to 6 minutes, until tender.
2 Add the flour and cook for 1 to 2 minutes, stirring constantly, then gradually add the broth and half the rosemary.
3 Bring to a boil and simmer for about 10 minutes, or until the mixture is halved in volume.
4 Check for seasoning and add the remaining rosemary.
5 Either cool to use later or serve with broiled meat immediately.

### serving suggestions
*Serve with any broiled or grilled meat or poultry.*

### storage
*The sauce may be kept in an airtight container and refrigerated for up to 2 days. Alternatively, the sauce may be frozen separately but, when reheating, it must come to a boil before serving.*

# pot roasted lamb shanks

Lamb is a great source of iron and zinc, and this recipe provides more than half your requirement for zinc and one quarter of your need for iron. Slow cooked in the oven, this pot roast will provide two servings for now and two, which can be frozen, for another time.

serves 4
preparation time 15 minutes
cooking time 2 hours

2 tablespoons vegetable oil
1 large onion, halved and sliced
3 large sticks of celery, cut into ¾ inch pieces
3 medium carrots, scrubbed and thickly sliced into chunks
2 medium lamb shanks (about 1 lb 10 oz)
1 teaspoon dried mixed herbs or 1 bouquet garni
3 bay leaves
1¾ cups water
¼ cup balsamic vinegar
2 tablespoons all-purpose flour

1 Preheat the oven to 325°F.
2 Heat the oil in a nonstick pan and add the onion, celery, and carrots. Cook over medium heat for about 5 minutes, or until they brown slightly. Remove the vegetables.
3 Adding a little more oil, if necessary, to the pan, then brown the lamb shanks over high heat for 2 to 3 minutes.
4 Put the lamb and vegetables into a ovenproof dish that has a lid and add the herbs. Pour 1½ cups water and the vinegar over the lamb, cover, and place in the oven for 1½ hours.
5 Remove from the oven. Mix the flour with ¼ cup water and stir into the stew to thicken.
6 Replace the lid on the dish and return to the oven for another 30 minutes, or until the vegetables are tender, the lamb is cooked through, and the sauce has thickened.
7 Remove the bay leaves and ease the meat away from the bone with a fork before serving.

serving suggestions
*Eat with* Leek Mashed Potatoes, *page 88, and a vitamin C-rich green vegetable, such as kale or broccoli.*

storage
*The cooked dish can be be kept in an airtight container and refrigerated for up to 2 days. Alternatively, it can be frozen for up to 3 months. Defrost overnight in a refrigerator before reheating until piping hot throughout.*

allergens
*Wheat (gluten), and celery.*

## MAKING A BOUQUET GARNI

*A delicious flavour enhancer and classic mix is thyme, bay leaf, parsley and celery. Wrap the herbs in the dark green part of a leek and tie tightly with string.*

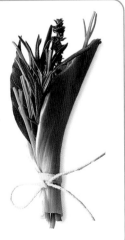

main dishes meats

# Moroccan lamb stew

Apricots and lamb make excellent partners in this spicy iron-rich casserole. The long cooking time makes the lamb really tender. This recipe will serve four to six, depending on your appetite, but leftovers can be frozen and eaten later if you're not serving all of it immediately.

serves 4 to 6
preparation time 15 minutes
cooking time 2½ hours

1 tablespoon olive oil
2 red onions, cut into lengthwise slices
2 cloves of garlic, crushed
1 lb 10 oz boneless lamb, such as shoulder, cubed
2 tablespoons ground cumin
1 cinnamon stick
2 bay leaves
2 small red chiles
2 cups water
2 heaping tablespoons tomato paste
1⅓ cups dried apricots

**to serve**
2 tablespoons chopped fresh cilantro
⅔ cup low-fat Greek yogurt (optional)

1 Preheat the oven to 325°F.
2 Heat the olive oil in a large, preferably nonstick, heavy saucepan or casserole that has a lid, add the onions and garlic, and sauté until the onion has softened.
3 Add the cubed lamb and cook, stirring, for 5 minutes, or until the lamb is lightly browned, adding a little more oil to prevent it from sticking, if necessary.
4 Add the spices and stir around, adding a little water, if needed, to prevent it from burning.
5 Pour in the rest of the water, the tomato paste, and apricots and stir well. Bring the ingredients slowly to the simmering point, then cover and transfer the pan or casserole to the oven to cook slowly about 2½ hours, or until the lamb is really tender.
6 Remove the cinnamon stick, bay leaves, and chile and sprinkle with the cilantro before serving.

**serving suggestions**
Eat with lowfat Greek yogurt accompanied by a simple green salad and couscous.

**storage**
The cooked dish can be refrigerated for 48 hours and will freeze well for up to 3 months. Thaw in the refrigerator overnight and reheat in a microwave until piping hot.

**allergens**
Milk (if served with yogurt).

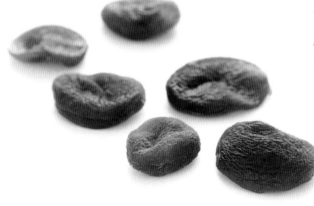

# lamb and green pepper kobabs with tzatziki

This lamb meatball-and-vegetable combination is full of pregnancy essentials, from immune-boosting vitamin C and zinc for you to essential vitamin $B_{12}$ for your baby. If you don't want to serve four, this recipe can be halved (you can freeze any leftover ground lamb from the package), or make up the mixture below and freeze in airtight bags for use another day.

serves  4
preparation time  10 minutes
cooking time  15 to 20 minutes

**for the lamb meatballs**
*2 slices whole wheat bread*
*1 small onion, peeled and quartered*
*1 lb ground lamb*
*2 cloves garlic, peeled*
*juice of ½ lime*
*1 tablespoon chopped cilantro*
*1 red chile, (optional), seeds removed and halved*
*black pepper*
*1 medium red onion, peeled and quartered*
*2 green bell peppers, seeds removed and cut into*
  *8 pieces each*

**to serve**
*Tzatziki, page 63*

1 Put the bread into a food processor and process until fine.
2 Add the onion, lamb, garlic, lime juice, cilantro, chile (if using), and black pepper and process until combined.
3 Transfer the mixture onto a clean cutting board and divide into 12.
4 Form each into a ball shape.
5 Preheat a broiler and lightly oil 4 skewers (wooden skewers need presoaking for 30 minutes in water).
6 Thread the onion and bell pepper pieces and lamb meatballs alternately on each skewer.
7 Line a baking sheet or the broiler tray with some aluminum foil  and place the kabobs on it.
8 Broil for 10 to 15 minutes, turning the kabobs often until the juices of the meatballs run clear.
9 Meanwhile prepare the tzatziki.

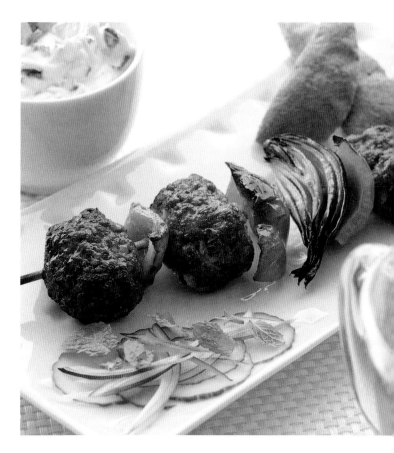

**serving suggestions**
*Eat with warm whole wheat pita bread and the Tzatziki.*

**storage**
*The cooked dish is not suitable for storage, but the meat mixture, prepared up through step 2, can be frozen in an airtight container for 1 month. Defrost in the refrigerator overnight and continue from step 3 of the recipe.*

**allergens**
*Milk (yogurt), gluten (bread).*

main dishes  meats

# crab linguine

When time is short, we often reach for pasta, but instead of a heavy creamy sauce, why not try this light sauce combining crab and asparagus with a little lemon boost. Asparagus is a great source of folic acid, but it is easily destroyed, so don't overcook it. If you prefer a different vegetable, slice a small trimmed leek, and, of course, you can always swap the crab for a can of tuna, although the latter contains little omega 3.

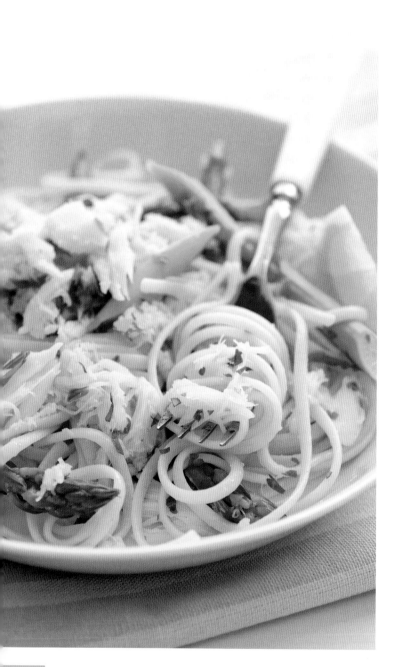

serves  1
preparation time  5 minutes
cooking time  15 minutes

*3 oz linguine or other long pasta*
*1 tablespoon olive oil*
*1 clove garlic*
*4 spears asparagus, trimmed into 1 inch slices*
*¼ cup dry white wine*
*3 oz mixed brown and white crab, canned or fresh*
*1 teaspoon lemon juice*
*1 tablespoon chopped parsley*

1 Cook the pasta according to the package directions.
2 Meanwhile, in a small saucepan, heat the oil, add the garlic and asparagus, and cook gently for 2 to 3 minutes without browning.
3 Add the wine and let simmer gently for about 5 minutes, until the asparagus is just tender. (The wine will be dealcoholized.)
4 Then add the crab, lemon juice, and parsley.
5 Drain the pasta and place in a serving bowl. Toss with the crab mixture and serve immediately.

## serving suggestions
*Accompany with a mixed salad.*

## allergens
*Wheat (gluten), shellfish.*

# crab cakes with watercress and orange salad

Crab is a good source of omega 3 fatty acids and iodine, with the brown meat containing much more than the white. The watercress and orange salad are served with a piquant dressing— all of which boosts the vitamin C and A content, too.

serves  2
preparation time  15 minutes
cooking time  15 minutes

¾ cup mashed potatoes
3½ oz crab, either canned or in a jar, brown, white, or mixed
2 scallions, finely chopped
1 tablespoon parsley, finely chopped
black pepper
1 tablespoon sesame seeds
1 large slice whole wheat bread or ½ cup fresh whole wheat bread crumbs
1 egg, beaten
vegetable oil for frying

for the salad
1 large orange, peeled and cut into sections
1½ bunches watercress, washed and trimmed into small sprigs

for the dressing
2 tablespoons freshly squeezed orange juice
1 tablespoon olive oil
1 tablespoon wine or sherry vinegar
pinch of sugar

## VARIATION
*You may want to swap the orange for pink grapefruit, and watercress for arugula. If you don't like crab, use flaked smoked mackerel.*

1 Put the mashed potatoes and crab into a bowl and add the onions and parsley. Stir to combine and divide into four equal portions. Shape each portion into a large patty, using flour, if necessary, to prevent it from sticking to your hands.
2 Process the bread to make crumbs and stir in the sesame seeds. Pour into a shallow bowl.
3 Beat the egg and pour into a shallow bowl.
4 Carefully dip each patty into the beaten egg, making sure it is covered, then lift into the bread crumbs. Pat these on so the patty's entire surface is covered before transferring it to a clean cutting board.
5 Heat 2 tablespoons oil in a nonstick skillet and cook the crab cakes, in batches if necessary, until the crumbs are golden on one side, then turn over and continue cooking until the cakes are piping hot through and golden brown on the outside.
6 Meanwhile, make the salad by combining the orange sections with the watercress and prepare the dressing by mixing together all the ingredients in a screw-top jar.
7 Pouring the dressing over the salad and serve the dressed salad with the hot crab cakes.

storage
*The crab cakes are best served immediately, but could be refrigerated before cooking for up to 24 hours in a airtight container. Once dressed, the salad must be eaten immediately.*

allergens
*Wheat (gluten), eggs, shellfish.*

# Greek-style tomato and white fish

An extremely simple and nutritious dinner dish, all this needs is a few new potatoes, or some crusty bread as an accompaniment. You can use any type of white fish. If you don't like the skin, ask the fish dealer to remove it for you, or use the technique described below.

serves  2
preparation time  5 minutes
cooking time  20 minutes

9 oz white fish fillet, such as red snapper, cod,
  halibut, flounder, or Alaskan pollock, washed
4 large ripe tomatoes
handful of basil leaves, torn
2 tablespoons Greek olive oil
black pepper, to taste

## FOOD SAFETY
*Use a separate board to prepare the raw fish. If you are using frozen fish, thaw it in the refrigerator and make sure it does not drip on other foods.*

1 Preheat the oven to 400°F.
2 Slice the tomatoes and lay in the bottom of an ovenproof container. Sprinkle with half of the basil leaves.
3 Skin the fish if you want or leave with the skin on. Dry with paper towels and fold in half. Place on top of the tomatoes and add the remaining basil.
4 Drizzle the oil on top, and grind over some black pepper.
5 Bake for 20 minutes or until the fish just flakes when prodded with a fork. Serve immediately, making sure to add all the cooking juices.

### serving suggestions
*Eat with new potatoes or crusty bread, and a side salad.*

### allergens
*Fish.*

## HOW TO SKIN A FLAT FISH
*You will need a sharp chef's knife and a clean cutting board. Lay the fish, skin side down, on the board, and press the tail end firmly with your fingers. Place the knife just beyond your fingers at a slight angle away from you and press instead of cut—you should go through the flesh but not the skin. Once you have made this cut, you should be able to push the knife away from you, using a sawing motion, if needed, as you hang onto the tail. The skin will "peel" away. If you accidentally cut through the flesh, just begin again from the other end.*

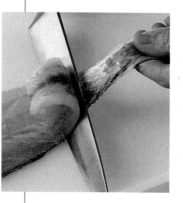

# potato-topped creamy fish casserole

This fish casserole is mild in flavor, high on nutrients, and goes down easily, making it a meal for days when you are a little run down. Later on in pregnancy, make a few to freeze when you are in the mood, so you have some available for when you are breastfeeding, because it provides plenty of calcium, too.

serves 4
preparation time 20 minutes
cooking time 20 to 25 minutes

2 cups lowfat milk
2 bay leaves
14 oz skinned white fish fillets, such as cod, halibut, red snapper, or Alaskan pollock
5 oz cooked shelled shrimp
2 tablespoons olive spread
¼ cup all-purpose flour
¼ cup light cream
⅔ cups frozen peas, thawed
1 tablespoon chopped parsley

for the mashed potato topping
6 Yukon gold or russet potatoes (about 1½ lb), peeled and quartered
1 or 2 tablespoons milk
pinch of salt (optional)

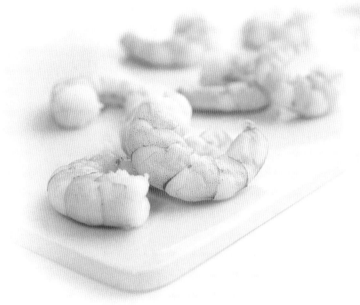

1 Preheat the oven to 350°F.
2 Pour the milk into a shallow saucepan or skillet and add the bay leaves and fish.
3 Heat gently to poach the fish, but do not let the milk to get too hot.
4 Meanwhile, prepare the mashed potatoes by steaming or boiling the potatoes until tender, then mashing with the milk and salt, if used.
5 Once the fish flakes easily when tested with a fork, carefully lift it out and spread out in an 8 x 8 inch lightly oiled ovenproof dish. Add the cooked shrimp.
6 Remove the bay leaves and drain the milk into a small bowl for use in the sauce.
7 Heat the spread in a saucepan and stir in the flour, cooking for 30 seconds or so before gradually adding the poaching milk, stirring constantly until the sauce has thickened.

8 Add the cream, peas, and parsley and pour the mixture over the fish, then spoon the potatoes over the top.
9 Bake for 25 to 30 minutes, until golden brown.

serving suggestions
*Accompany with additional peas or a few carrots.*

storage
*The cooked dish can be kept in an airtight container and refrigerated for 24 hours. Alternatively, it may be frozen for up to 3 months at the end of step 9. Keep it in its dish and wrap with plastic wrap or aluminum foil. Defrost in the refrigerator overnight and cook as in stage 10, allowing a little longer. It must be piping hot when served.*

allergens
*Fish, shellfish.*

main dishes seafood

113

# sea bass with pomegranate salsa

Cooking fish "en papillote" is a fantastic way of preserving moisture and minimizing fishy cooking odors. Sea bass is a white fish rich in the B vitamins, especially $B_3$ and $B_{12}$, and also contains bone building calcium. Here, it is served with a salsa containing pomegranate seeds, which are rich in protective polyphenols.

serves  2
preparation time  10 minutes
cooking time  20 minutes

2 (5 oz) fillets sea bass
1 garlic clove, crushed
1 teaspoon grated ginger root
1 teaspoon grated lime zest

### for the pomegranate salsa
½ teaspoon grated ginger root
½ teaspoon grated lime zest
1 teaspoon fresh cilantro (optional)
1 teaspoon honey
2 teaspoons olive oil
1 teaspoon lemon juice
½ cup pomegranate seeds

1 Preheat the oven to 375°F.
2 Cut two pieces of parchment paper or aluminum foil, each about 12 inches square. Lightly oil the foil, if using.
3 Lay each fish fillet on a piece of parchment or foil and sprinkle with the garlic, ginger, and lime zest.
4 Fold over the top and sides of the parchment or foil loosely to make a package and put onto a baking sheet.
5 Cook for 15 to 20 minutes, or until the fish flakes easily when tested with a fork.
6 Meanwhile, mix together all the ingredients for the salsa in a small bowl.
7 Carefully transfer the fish to a warm plate and serve immediately with the salsa.

### serving suggestions
*Accompany with* Gratin of Potato, *page 139 or new potatoes, and a seasonal green vegetable.*

### storage
*The cooked dish is not suitable for storage, but the salsa may be kept in an airtight container and refrigerated for up to 2 days. Neither is suitable for freezing.*

### allergens
*Contains: fish.*

# salmon and asparagus en croûte

Salmon (or trout) is full of pregnancy essentials, especially omega 3s and vitamin D. This particularly easy recipe uses phyllo pasty to wrap the fish, and if you add in a few asparagus tips, you'll be getting a little folic acid, too.

serves  1
preparation time  5 minutes
cooking time  20 minutes

*2 sheets of phyllo pastry*
*a little vegetable oil or an oil mister*
*2 or 3 spears of asparagus*
*3½ oz skinless fillet of salmon or trout*
*few drops lemon or lime juice (optional)*

1 Preheat the oven to 375°F.
2 Place one sheet of pastry on a clean surface and either brush or spray with oil.
3 Put the fish in the center and place the asparagus, trimmed to the same size as the fillet, on top.
4 Sprinkle with the lemon juice, if using, and wrap up the package, tucking the ends under.
5 Lightly brush or spray the other sheet of phyllo with oil and place the package in the middle; roll up the pastry. Transfer the package to a baking sheet and spray or brush again with oil.
6 Bake for 20 minutes or until the package is golden brown. Serve immediately.

### serving suggestions
*Accompany with some boiled new potatoes and seasonal vegetables. Add a few more steamed asparagus stems for more folic acid. You may also want to accompany with* Piquant Avocado Dip, *page 66,* Lime Dressing, *page 119, or* Tzatziki, *page 63.*

### allergens
*Wheat (gluten), fish.*

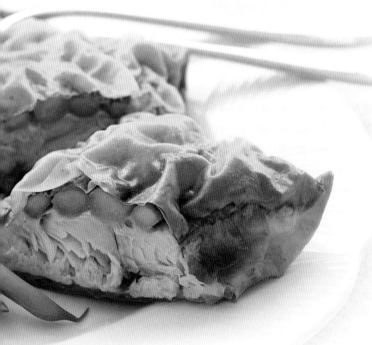

> **COOK'S TIP**
> *When wrapping a phyllo pastry package using two sheets of pastry, place the filling on the first sheet and wrap, tucking the ends under. Then place the package on the second sheet and wrap so the tucked-under ends of the second sheet are opposite those of the first.*

<salmon and asparagus en croûte
with piquant avocado dip

# smoked salmon flakes with herbed lentils

This simple, warm dish uses cooked lentils for speed, and makes a delicious lunch or light dinner dish. It provides one third of your day's needs for iron and zinc as well as gives you a great boost of omega 3 and vitamin D.

serves  2
preparation time  10 minutes
cooking time  5 minutes

1 large stick celery, finely chopped
1¼ cups cooked lentils
1 cup arugula leaves, coarsely chopped
12 sprigs of watercress, coarsely chopped
5½ oz hot smoked salmon, skinned and flaked

**for the dressing**
½ cup reduced fat crème fraiche
1 tablespoon horseradish sauce
juice of ½ lemon
grated zest of ½ lemon

1 Put the celery into a small saucepan of boiling water and cook for 3 to 4 minutes to just soften. Drain.
2 Warm the lentils in a microwave oven or in a saucepan with 1 tablespoon water to prevent them from sticking. Stir in the celery. Drain, if required, before mixing in the arugula and watercress.
3 Make the dressing by combining all the ingredients in a small bowl.
4 Stir the dressing into the lentil mixture and then add the salmon flakes. Serve immediately.

**serving suggestions**
Eat with a few cherry tomatoes and, if hungry, a slice of whole wheat bread.

**storage**
The cooked dish is not suitable for storage, but the sauce may be kept in an airtight container and refrigerated for up to 2 days. Alternatively, the sauce may be frozen separately but, when reheating, it must come to a boil before serving.

**allergens**
Fish, milk (crème fraîche), celery.

# sardines with avocado and cherry tomatoes

As a sustainable, oil-rich fish, sardines are a great choice in pregnancy. Because the bones are small and soft, they are normally eaten, which provides you with essential calcium, and they are also an especially rich source of vitamin D.

serves  2
preparation time  15 minutes
cooking time  10 minutes

**for the sardines**
*14 oz fresh sardines*
*1 tablespoon flour*
*1 teaspoon paprika*
*vegetable oil for frying*

**for the avocado and cherry tomato salad**
*1 medium Hass avocado*
*juice of ½ lemon or lime*
*8 cherry tomatoes*
*1 tablespoon chopped parsley*

1 Firstly, wash the sardines and with a sharp knife remove the head and tail. Slit open from the head end to remove the insides and discard. Wash again and pat dry on paper towels. Continue until all the sardines are cleaned and prepared.
2 Make the salad by chopping the peeled avocado into cubes, tossing in the lemon juice, and mixing with the cherry tomatoes and parsley.
3 Place the flour on a shallow plate and mix in the paprika. Dip each fish in a little seasoned flour.
4 Heat a couple tablespoons oil in a nonstick skillet, and when hot, fry the sardines for 4 to 5 minutes, turning half way through, until they are tender but slightly crispy. Serve immediately with the avocado and tomato salad.

**serving suggestions**
*Eat with whole wheat bread as a light dinner or lunch.*

**allergens**
*Wheat (gluten), fish.*

# tuna and vegetable pasta casserole

Pasta and cans of tuna and tomatoes are great pantry staples. Liven then up with vitamin C-rich bell peppers and basil to make this nutritious dish that is quick and easy to prepare.

serves  4
preparation time  15 minutes
cooking time  35 minutes

1 tablespoon olive oil
1 medium onion, coaresly chopped
2 cloves garlic, crushed
2 medium red bell peppers, quartered and sliced crosswise
5 oz pasta shapes
1 (14½ oz) can diced tomatoes in juice
handful of basil leaves
2 (5 oz) cans tuna in oil, drained
black pepper, optional
1 cup shredded cheddar cheese

1 Heat the oil in a large nonstick saucepan and sauté the onion and garlic for 5 minutes until just translucent. Stir in the bell peppers and cover and cook for another few minutes until the bell peppers are softened.
2 Meanwhile, cook the pasta according to the package directions.
3 Add the canned tomatoes to the vegetable mix and bring to a boil. Turn down the heat, cover, and simmer for 5 minutes.
4 Remove from the heat and stir in the basil leaves and drained tuna. Grind over a little black pepper.
5 When the pasta has cooked, drain and transfer to a large ovenproof dish. Cover with the sauce, mix slightly to combine, and sprinkle with the shredded cheese.
6 Place in a preheated oven for 20 to 25 minutes, or until the cheese is golden brown and the casserole is piping hot. Serve immediately.

## serving suggestions
*Eat with steamed broccoli or cauliflower or a large green salad.*

## storage
*The pasta dish can be prepared up to the end of step 5 and chilled for 24 hours or frozen for up to 2 months. Then defrost in the refrigerator and cook as in step 6. If you prefer to freeze the cooked dish, then defrost it in the refrigerator and reheat in a microwave until it is piping hot.*

## allergens
*Wheat (gluten), fish, milk (cheese).*

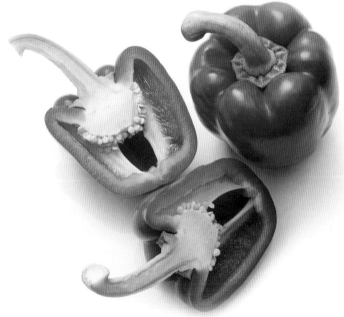

# tuna steaks with sun-dried tomato crust and lime dressing

Oven cooked with a simple bread crumb and tomato topping and lime dressing, this fresh tuna meal is a great source of omega 3 fatty acids and supplies all your vitamin D needs for a day.

serves 2
preparation time  15 minutes
cooking time  20 to 25 minutes

*1 large slice whole wheat bread*
*½ cup drained sun-dried tomatoes in oil*
*1 clove garlic*
*few basil leaves*
*2 (5½ oz) tuna steaks*

### for the lime dressing
*2 rounded tablespoons fat-reduced sour cream or*
  *crème fraîche*
*2 rounded tablespoons lowfat Greek yogurt*
*1 teaspoon grated lime zest*
*2 teaspoons lime juice*

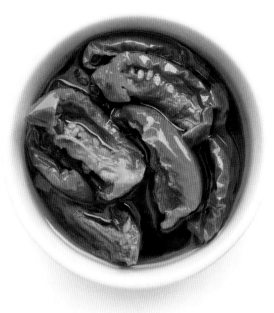

1 Preheat the oven to 350°F.
2 Put the bread, tomatoes, basil, and oil into a food processor or blender and blend until fine.
3 Wipe the tuna with clean paper towels,  place on a lightly oiled baking sheet, and carefully press half the bread crumb mixture onto each steak.
4 Bake for 20 minutes, or until the tuna flakes easily when tested with a fork.
5 Meanwhile, make the lime dressing by combining all the ingredients in a small bowl.
6 Serve the hot tuna with the dressing.

### serving suggestions
*Accompany with new potatoes and peas, snow peas, green beans, or a mixed salad.*

### storage
*The cooked dish is not suitable for storage, but the sauce may be kept in an airtight container and refrigerated for up to 2 days.*

### allergens
*Fish, gluten, milk (creams/ yogurt).*

main dishes seafood

# stuffed portobello mushrooms

These flat, dark, open-capped mushrooms are ideal for stuffing, and the simple mixture used here is prepared in a flash. The resulting dish provides a host of the B vitamins and calcium, all of which are essential for your developing baby.

serves  2
preparation time  5 minutes
cooking time  35 minutes

2 large portobello mushrooms
2 large slices whole wheat bread, torn into pieces
2 cloves garlic
1 cup drained sun-dried tomatoes in oil
½ cup reduced fat shredded cheddar cheese

1 Preheat the oven to 375°F.
2 Wipe the cap and stem of each mushroom with damp paper towels and remove the stem.
3 Put the stems, garlic, and bread into a food processor and blend until fine.
4 Add the tomatoes and pulse to coarsely chop.

5 Press this mixture into the mushrooms and place them on a lightly oiled baking sheet.
6 Sprinkle the cheese over the mushrooms and bake for 30 to 35 minutes, until the mushrooms are tender and the cheese is melted and turning golden.

## serving suggestions
*Eat with a green salad for lunch, or add baked or new potatoes and roasted vegetables for a delicious light dinner dish.*

## allergens
*Wheat (gluten).*

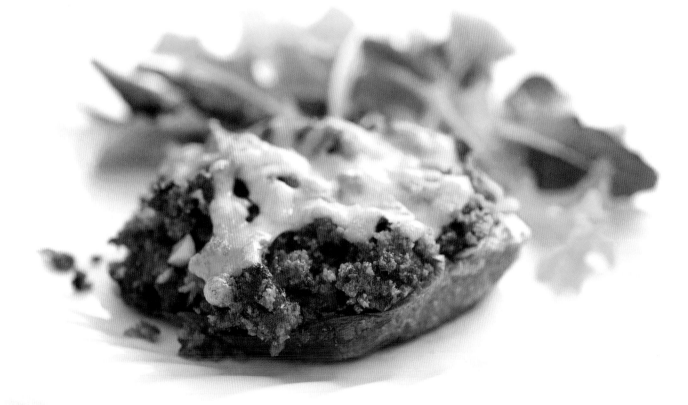

# butternut squash casserole with halloumi and pomegranate

This is a great fall and winter meal when squash are plentiful. It provides more than three times your vitamin A needs, and is low in sodium, so dig in. Pomegranates contain many protective antioxidants and, from Biblical times, have been regarded as one of nature's most "powerful" fruits. Recent studies indicate they may help lower blood pressure, thus reducing your risk of preeclampsia.

serves  2 to 3
preparation time  15 minutes
cooking time  30 to 35 minutes

*1 onion, coarsely chopped*
*1 tablespoon vegetable oil*
*½ butternut squash, peeled and cut into ¾ inch cubes*
*1 sweet potato, peeled and cubed*
*¼ cup water*
*5 cups frozen leaf spinach, thawed*
*3½ oz halloumi or feta, coarsely grated or chopped*
*seeds from one small pomegranate (about ½ cup)*

1 Preheat the oven to 375°F.
2 Heat the oil in a large ovenproof saucepan with a lid and gently sauté the onion for 5 minutes, until just softening.
3 Add the cubes of squash and sweet potato, stir, and cover. Reduce the heat to low and let the vegetables cook for 5 minutes, stirring occasionally to prevent it from sticking.
4 Pour in the water, replace the lid, and place the pan in the oven for 20 to 25 minutes, or until the vegetables are just tender, adding a little more water, if necessary.
5 Stir in the spinach and sprinkle with the halloumi. Return the pan to the oven for 10 minutes, or until the cheese is melted and starting to brown.
6 Sprinkle with the pomegranate seeds.

### serving suggestions
*This is a meal in itself, but if you want, add an arugula and watercress salad.*

### storage
*The cooked dish minus the pomegranate seeds can be stored in an airtight container and refrigerated for up to 24 hours. Reheat until piping hot throughout in a microwave oven, then serve sprinkled with the seeds.*

### allergens
*Milk (cheese).*

## COOK'S TIP
*Look for prepared squash and sweet potato cubes to save you time in the kitchen.*

## VARIATION
*For a spicier dish, add 2 teaspoons toasted cumin seeds at the end of step 2, when the onions are soft and/or a little chili powder to the vegetables in step 3.*

main dishes  vegetarian

# creamy vegetarian ground "beef"

Vegetarian textured soy protein makes an easy dinner dish that vegetarians and carnivores alike will enjoy, and that can also be frozen. The addition of peanut butter gives it a creamy texture, and adds antioxidant vitamin E and copper, an essential mineral for the functioning of the vascular system.

serves 4
preparation time 10 minutes
cooking time 20 minutes

1 tablespoon olive oil
1 onion, finely chopped
1 clove garlic, crushed
1 small green bell pepper, diced
1 teaspoons ground cumin
10 oz vegetarian textured soy protein
2 tablespoons tomato paste
1¾ cups water
3 tablespoons peanut butter

1 Heat the oil in a saucepan with a lid and gently sauté the onion and garlic for 5 minutes, or until just softening.
2 Add the green bell pepper and cumin and continue to sauté for another minute or so.
3 Stir in the textured protein and tomato paste.
4 Pour in the water and bring the mixture to a boil.
5 Stir, cover, and reduce heat. Simmer the mixture for 15 minutes, stirring occasionally, and adding more water, if the mixture seems dry.
6 Stir in the peanut butter and serve.

### serving suggestions
*Eat with rice and a green vegetable or use as a filling for a baked potato and accompany with a salad.*

### storage
*This may be kept in an airtight container and refrigerated for 2 days or frozen for 2 months. Thaw in the refrigerator and reheat until piping hot throughout in a microwave oven.*

### allergens
*Peanuts.*

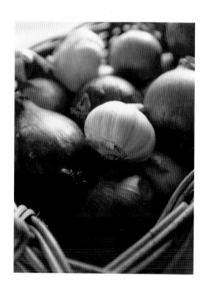

### VARIATION
*For a spicier mix, add ½ teaspoon chili powder and additional cumin in step 2 and 2 teaspoons garam masala and 1 tablespoon chopped cilantro before serving.*

# pasta primavera

This quick, tasty dish provides two servings of vegetables, plenty of fiber, and 50 percent of your pregnancy requirement of vitamin C. By using whole-grain pasta, you will also increase the amount of iron in this meal to one third of your needs.  If you are struggling with nausea, the simple fresh tomato sauce made without onion or garlic can make it easier for you to be in the kitchen.

serves 2
preparation time  5 minutes
cooking time  20 minutes

2 large ripe tomatoes
1 tablespoon olive oil
8 oz dry whole-grain fusilli or other pasta shape
1 cup tiny broccoli florets
½ cup trimmed green bean pieces (¾ inch pieces)
½ cup finely sliced snow peas

### to serve
2 tablespoons grated Parmesan or pecorino cheese
and black pepper

1 Skin the tomatoes, cut into quarters, and scoop out the seeds. Coarsely chop.
2 Heat the olive oil in a saucepan and add the tomato. Cover and cook gently for 15 to 20 minutes, stirring occasionally until the tomato flesh is really soft.
3 Whilst the sauce is cooking, boil a large saucepan of water and cook the pasta according to the package directions, adding the broccoli and green beans and for the last 3 to 4 minutes and the snow peas for the final minute.
4 Drain the pasta and vegetables and divide between 2 serving dishes, then and pour the sauce over them.
5 Grind black pepper over the pasta, sprinkle with the cheese, and serve.

### storage
*The cooked dish is not suitable for storage, but the sauce may be kept in an airtight container and refrigerated for up to 2 days or frozen. When reheating the sauce, make sure it comes to the boil before serving.*

### allergens
*Wheat (gluten), milk (cheese).*

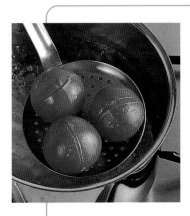

### HOW TO SKIN TOMATOES
*Score a cross in the bottom of the tomato and place in a heatproof bowl. Pour  boiling water over it and let stand for a minute. Then lift out with a slotted spoon and, using a sharp knife, peel off the skin.*

### VARIATION
*If you prefer to use fresh pasta, cook for the recommended time on the package and steam the vegetables separately. You may want to add a few torn fresh basil leaves to the sauce.*

# roasted baby vegetables with tofu

Silken or firm tofu is made from soybeans and is a versatile food, low in fat and high in protein. It is also a good source of calcium, so if you can't tolerate dairy foods, it makes a good alternative to cheese.

serves 2 to 3
preparation time 10 minutes
cooking time 45 minutes

*10½ oz firm tofu*
*1 tablespoon vegetable oil*
*1 teaspoon soy sauce*
*7 oz baby eggplants*
*1 red bell pepper*
*1 red onion*
*1 small zucchini or 2 baby zucchini*
*2 tablespoons olive oil*
*a few sprigs of thyme, optional*

1 Preheat the oven to 400°F.
2 Cut the tofu into large cubes and marinate in the vegetable oil and soy sauce for 10 minutes.
3 Meanwhile, prepare the vegetables. Quarter the eggplants, cut the red bell pepper into slices, slice the red onion lengthwise, and halve or quarter the zucchini.
4 Pour the olive oil into a roasting pan. Add the vegetables and toss them in the oil, making sure they are well coated.
5 Bake 40 minutes or until the vegetables are tender.

*serving suggestions*
*Accompany with Almond Rice (page 136), couscous, or tabbouleh.*

**allergens**
*Soy.*

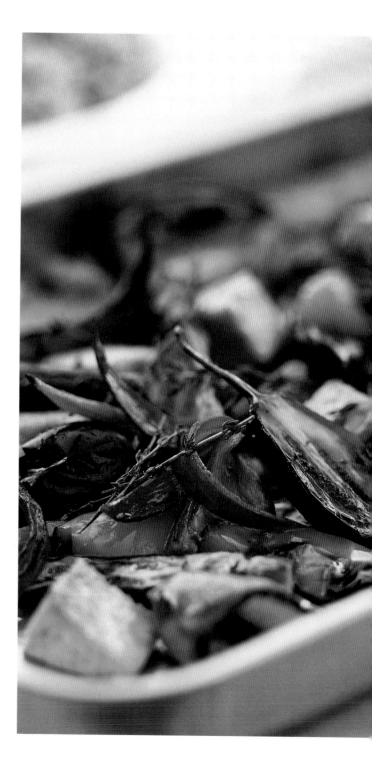

# vegetable crepes with red pepper sauce

Although it has a long list of ingredients, this nutritious meal is worth making up as a double or triple batch of the crepes and/or the red pepper sauce to freeze for later use. You can also use tortilla wraps. The complete recipe provides a fantastic boost of vitamin A, as well as supplying more than 50 percent of your needed calcium and vitamin C.

serves  2 (makes 4 to 6 pancakes depending on the
    size of your pan)
preparation time  30 minutes
cooking time  30 minutes

### for the pancakes
*½ cup whole wheat flour*
*½ cup white all-purpose flour*
*1 extra-large egg*
*1 tablespoon olive oil*
*1 cup lowfat milk*
*1 tablespoon vegetable oil, for cooking*

### for the red pepper sauce
*1 tablespoon vegetable oil*
*1 onion, finely chopped*
*1 red bell pepper, seeded and coarsely chopped*
*1 (14½ oz) can diced tomatoes in juice*

### for the vegetables
*1 tablespoon vegetable oil*
*1 leek, trimmed, sliced in half lengthwise, then cut
    into semicircles*
*1 carrot, finely diced*
*⅔ cup frozen edamame (soybeans)*
*⅔ cup frozen corn kernels*

*½ cup shredded reduced fat cheddar cheese*

1 Prepare the crepes. Put all the ingredients into a blender and process until smooth. You should have a pouring batter; if it is too thick add a little more milk or water. Let stand.

2 Prepare the red pepper sauce. Heat the oil in a nonstick saucepan and, over low heat, gently sauté the onion until just softened. Add the bell pepper and cook gently for 5 minutes, stirring occasionally.

Pour in the tomatoes, and simmer, covered, for 10 to 15 minutes. or until the vegetables are softened.

3 Meanwhile, in another nonstick saucepan, heat the oil for the vegetable filling and gently cook the carrot and leek over low heat for 10 to 15 minutes, or until tender. Use a lid to cover and stir occasionally. Stir in the frozen beans and corn and continue cooking over low heat until all the vegetables are cooked through.

4 To cook the crepes, put the 1 tablespoon of vegetable oil in small cup or egg cup and preferably use a nonstick skillet. For each pancake, heat the pan then pour in a dribble of oil. When the oil is hot, pour in some batter, swirling it around to thinly cover the bottom of the pan. Cook until lightly browned on one side, then flip over to cook the reverse. Keep the pancakes warm under aluminum foil while preparing the other ones.

5 When you are ready to serve, fill 2 crepes per person with the vegetable mixture and place on a warm plate. Spoon some red pepper sauce over the crepes and sprinkle with some cheese. Serve immediately.

### serving suggestions
*You may want to place the crepes in a serving dish, cover with the sauce and cheese, then bake for 10–15 minutes, until the cheese browns.*

### storage
*The pancakes can be frozen individually layered between wax paper or plastic wrap. The red pepper sauce can also be frozen in an airtight contain and defrosted in the refrigerator overnight. Alternatively, the whole stuffed crepes may be frozen in an freezer to oven dish so that they can be reheated at a later date.*

### allergens
*Wheat (gluten), eggs, milk, and cheese.*

# black-eyed pea, dried currant, and fresh mint stew

This has to be one of the easiest and most healthy dishes for early in pregnancy. Black-eyed peas are peculiarly high in folate, and even allowing for nutrient loss in cooking, one serving of this dish will provide 45 percent of your dietary needs. The stew also has great credentials for its iron content, and for bone-building phosphorus. An all round winner.

serves  2
preparation time  5 minutes
cooking time  20 minutes

1 tablespoon olive oil
1 onion, coarsely chopped
2 sticks of celery, finely sliced
2 cloves garlic
1 (15 oz) can of black-eyed peas in water, rinsed
  and drained
1 teaspoon cumin
¼ cup dried currants
about 1 cup water
1 tablespoon freshly chopped mint
black pepper

1 Heat the oil in a nonstick saucepan and gently sauté the onion, celerly, and garlic until softened.
2 Add the beans, cumin, and currants and stir in almost all the water.
3 Bring to a boil, stir, and cover. Reduce the heat to simmering point and cook for 15 minutes, or until the vegetables are just tender, adding more water, if required.
4 Remove from the heat and stir in the mint and season to taste.

## serving suggestions
*Eat with rice, pearl barley, or couscous, and  a green vegetable or sliced tomatoes.*

## storage
*The cooked dish will freeze for up to 3 months, or can be kept in the refrigerator for 48 hours.*

## allergens
*Celery.*

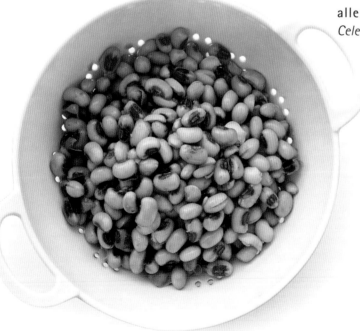

# sweet potato and chestnut jalousie

This wonderful party dish, based on a recipe by the well-known chef Tony Turnbull, is good for you as well as tasty for any vegetarian guests. It is high in vitamin A, and provides more than 50 percent of your pregnancy needs for copper.

serves  4 to 6
preparation time  30 minutes
cooking time  45 minutes plus 30 to 35 minutes

**for the roasted vegetables**
½ butternut squash, peeled and cut into cubes
2 to 3 sweet potatoes (about 1 lb), peeled and cut into cubes
2 tablespoons olive oil

**for the remaining filling**
1 tablespoon vegetable oil
1 onion, finely chopped
9 oz button mushrooms, wiped and quartered
7 oz vacuum packed unsweetened whole chestnuts, left whole or if large, halved
2 teaspoons ground cumin
3 tablespoons flour
1¾ cups vegetable broth or water
1 tablespoon mushroom ketchup
2 tablespoons parsley, coarsely chopped

**for the pastry**
1 (1 lb) package puff pastry
beaten egg to glaze

1   Preheat the oven to 400°F.
2   Put the sweet potato and butternut squash cubes into a clean plastic bag and pour in the olive oil. Shake to coat with the oil and transfer to a baking sheet. Roast for 35 to 45 minutes, or until the vegetables are tender. Let  cool; don't turn off the oven.
3   To prepare the remaining filling, heat the oil in a nonstick saucepan and gently sauté the onion until soft, then add the mushrooms. Cover and cook for 5 minutes, or until they are softened a little.
4   Stir in the cumin, then the chestnuts.

5   Sprinkle with the flour and stir to coat the vegetables. Pour in a little broth to make a thick sauce, then add the remaining broth and the ketchup. Bring to a boil to thicken the sauce, then remove the vegetable mixture from the heat and let cool slightly.
6   To prepare the pastry, sprinkle some flour on a clean work surface and cut the pastry in half. Roll out each pastry half as thinly as you can, making two rectangles, one slightly larger than the other but both about 8 x 12 inches.
7   Place the smaller rectangle of pastry on a lined baking sheet.
8   Mix together the cooled squash and sweet potato with the mushroom mixture and add the parsley. Spoon onto the pastry rectangle on the baking sheet, leaving a 1 inch border all around. Brush this border with water.
9   Using a sharp knife, cut diagonal slashes in the other pastry rectangle, leaving a 1 inch border around the edge. Pick up the pastry on a rolling pin and place on top of the filling. Press the border edges together, trimming off any extra pastry.
10  Brush lightly with the beaten egg and bake for 30 to 35 minutes until the pastry is risen and golden.

## serving suggestions
*Because of the double cooking method, there is little vitamin C in this dish so serve with steamed broccoli or snow peas, or a watercress and orange salad.*

## storage
*For best results, serve immediately, but the cooked dish may be refrigerated for 48 hours in an airtight container, and reheated in a conventional oven until piping hot.*

## allergens
*Wheat (gluten), eggs, nuts.*

# tarka dhal

My version of this Indian classic is healthy comfort food. Lentils or dried peas are a good source of iron, as are the curry spices.

serves 4
preparation time 5 minutes
cooking time 30 minutes

1½ cups red lentils, washed
3 cups cold water
5 cardamon pods
2 bay leaves
2 tablespoons vegetable oil
1 onion, finely chopped
3 cloves garlic, crushed
1 teaspoon ground cumin
1 teaspoon ground turmeric
2 teaspoons ground coriander
pinch of salt
black pepper

1 Put the lentils into a saucepan and cover with the water. Add the bay leaves and cardamom pods and bring to a boil. Stir, reduce the heat, and let simmer for about 30 minutes, until the lentils are softened, adding more water, if required.
2 Meanwhile, in a separate saucepan, heat the oil and sauté the onion and garlic until softened.
3 Add the cumin, turmeric, and coriander and cook for a minute before removing the pan from the heat.
4 When the lentils are cooked, stir in the fried onions, season to taste, remove the bay leaves, and serve.

### serving suggestions
*To add some spice, add 1 tablespoon each garam marsala and chopped cilantro before serving. Eat with* Almond Rice *(page 136), sliced tomatoes, and a green vegetable.*

### storage
*The dahl can be refrigerated in an airtight container for 2 days or frozen for 2 months. Thaw well at room temperature and reheat until piping hot.*

# water chestnut and cashew nut stir fry

Cashew nuts may seem an unlikely source of iron, but even a small portion provides you with a good supply of the mineral. Iron absorption is facilitated by the vitamin C supplied by the bell peppers, making this quick dish a pregnancy winner.

serves 2
preparation time 5 minutes
cooking time 10 minutes

½ cup plain cashew nuts
2 plain noodle nests (about 3 oz each)
1 tablespoon canola oil
½ cup drained and sliced water chestnuts
10 oz package prepared mixed bell peppers (about 2 cups)
1 or 2 tablespoons water
1 tablespoon dry sherry
2 teaspoons reduced sodium soy sauce

1 Toast the cashew nuts in an oven preheated to 400°F for a few minutes until lightly browned, or dry fry in a nonstick saucepan over low heat.
2 Meanwhile, put the dry noodle nests into a heatproof bowl, pour boiling water over them, and let stand for 5 minutes, or prepare according to package directions.
3 Heat the oil in a wok or large skillet, preferably nonstick, and stir-fry the water chestnuts and vegetable mixture for 4 to 5 minutes, adding a little water if they begin to stick to the pan.
4 Stir in the cooked noodles, sherry, and soy sauce and once combined, sprinkle with the cashew nuts.

### allergens
*Wheat (gluten), nuts (cashews).*

# brazil nut burgers

This recipe is both simple and versatile—you can use different types of nuts or breads
for a change of pace.

serves  4
preparation time  5 minutes
cooking time  30 minutes

*²/₃ cup Brazil nuts*
*2 large scallions, chopped*
*2 slices white bread*
*1 egg, separated*
*1 red bell pepper, diced*
*salt and black pepper, to taste*
*oil, for greasing*

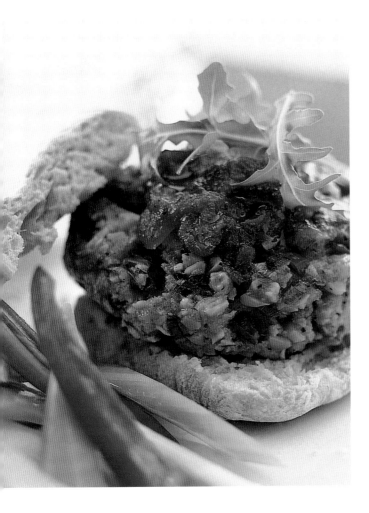

1 Preheat the oven to 350°F.
2 Put the Brazil nuts, scallions, and bread into a food
  processor and process until well chopped.
3 Add the egg yolk and red bell pepper and mix well.
4 Season to taste. If the mixture needs more liquid to
  bind it, add the egg white.
5 Form the mixture into 4 even balls and press down
  to form patties about 1 inch thick.
6 Place the patties on a greased baking sheet and cook
  for 25 to 30 minutes, or until the burgers are slightly
  browned and crunchy on the outside.

## serving suggestions
*Serve in a toasted bun with some tomato relish and a
side salad or baked new potatoes.*

## storage
*The cooked burgers can be frozen once cold, and reheated
until piping hot in the microwave.*

## allergens
*Gluten (wheat), eggs, nuts (Brazils).*

> **VARIATION**
> *Use ciabatta rolls instead of burger buns for a change.
> Warm them in the oven first to crisp up the crust.*

# kachumbari

This vitamin C-rich salad from East Africa is a great accompaniment to broiled meat. The key to making a success of this salad is a sharp knife or mandoline slicer, because everything needs to be sliced finely.

serves  4
preparation time  10 minutes
cooking time  0 minutes

*3 or 4 large ripe tomatoes*
*1 small green bell pepper*
*1 small red onion*
*pinch of salt*
*juice of 1 small lemon (about 4 teaspoons)*
*1 tablespoon chopped cilantro*

1 Wash the tomatoes and slice as finely as you can.
2 Remove the stem and seeds from the bell pepper, quarter, and slice finely.
3 Peel the onion, halve, and slice finely.
4 Mix the 3 vegetables in a bowl with a pinch of salt and pour the lemon juice over them.
5 Stir in the cilantro, cover, and chill for at least 15 minutes to let the salt draw some of the juices from the salad vegetables.

## serving suggestions
*Use to accompany broiled meats or steaks of all kinds.*

## storage
*The salad may be kept in an airtight container and refrigerated for 24 hours.*

# two pear salad

This cool salad will make a welcome change from cooked vegetables in the winter months, when pear and avocado are widely available. The avocado provides healthy monounsaturated fats as well as vitamin E.

serves  2
preparation time  10 minutes
cooking time  0 minutes

**for the dressing**
*1 tablespoon honey*
*2 tablespoons olive oil*
*grated zest of one lime*
*1 tablespoon lime juice*

**for the salad**
*1 ripe avocado pear*
*1 large ripe pear, such as Bosc*
*1 cup shredded romaine lettuce*

1 Make the dressing by whisking together all the ingredients in a large bowl.
2 Peel the avocado, remove the pit, and cut into cubes. Stir into the dressing to prevent them from browning.
3 Cut the other pear into quarters, and remove the core. Cube and add to the bowl. If the skin is tough, you may want to peel it first.
4 Put the shredded lettuce into a serving dish.
5 Spoon the pears and dressing over the lettuce and serve immediately.

## serving suggestions
*Use to accompany broiled poultry, or add a handful of toasted walnuts and serve with bread as a main dish.*

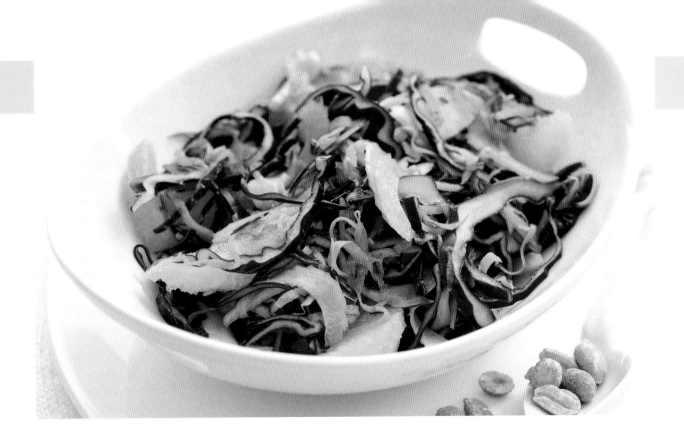

# ginger and orange slaw

A tangy salad containing ginger to help combat nausea, this slaw utilizes winter produce with its high vitamin C content to keep winter bugs at bay. Enjoy it with baked potatoes, cold meat (including leftover turkey), or on its own with a few added nuts.

serves 3
preparation time 10 minutes
cooking time 0 minutes

¾ inch piece fresh ginger root, finely grated
1 tablespoon lemon juice
1 tablespoon honey
¼ small red cabbage (about 1½ cups when prepared)
1 stick of celery, washed and trimmed
1 large carrot, peeled
1 large orange

1 Mix the grated ginger, lemon juice, and honey together in a large mixing bowl.
2 Using a mandoline slicer or food processor, finely slice the cabbage and celery and stir into the bowl.
3 Coarsely grate the carrot and add to the other ingredients.
4 Using a small sharp knife, peel the orange. Then hold the orange above the bowl to catch any drips, and cut away the flesh of each section, halve, and add to the salad.
5 Stir all the ingredients together well and serve, or cover with plastic wrap and chill until required.

**serving suggestions**
*Great with roasted chicken thighs and a baked potato; or add a few dry roasted peanuts and have as a snack.*

**storage**
*The salad will keep refrigerated for 24 hours in an airtight container.*

**allergens**
*Celery.*

vegetables and side dishes

# curly kale with garlic cherry tomatoes

Curly kale is an often overlooked vegetable, rich in vitamins A and C, which will help boost your immune system and keep "bugs" at bay. If you haven't tried this vegetable before, prepare this simple recipe and you'll be suprised at how delicious it can be.

serves  2
preparation time  5 minutes
cooking time  15 minutes

1 tablespoon olive oil
8 cherry tomatoes, washed and halved
2 gloves garlic, crushed
2 cups coarsely chopped curly kale
black pepper

1 Heat the oil in a small saucepan and gently cook the tomatoes and garlic, stirring frequently.
2 Meanwhile, wash and drain the curly kale.
3 When the tomatoes are softened, add the kale to the pan, stir well, and bring to a boil. Let simmer for a few minutes until the kale has wilted and is just tender.
4 Remove from the heat, grind some black pepper over the salad, and serve immediately

### serving suggestions
*Good as an accompaniment to broiled meat or poultry.*

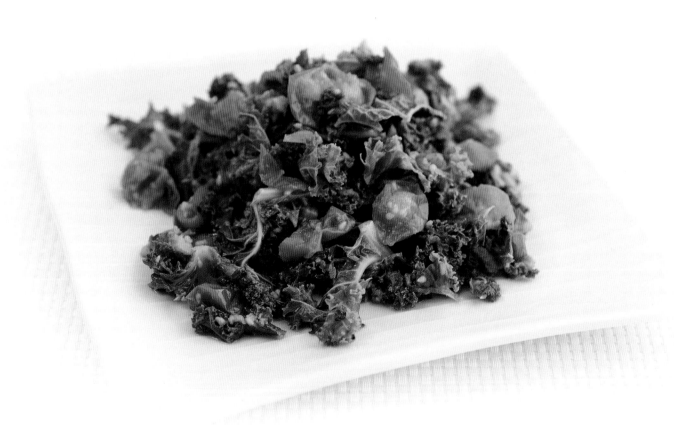

# broccoli with almonds

Look for purple baby broccoli at the farmer's market (or grown your own)—it is a fantastically good source of folate, which is especially important in early pregnancy. Out of season, use regular broccoli, remembering to steam it till just tender to preserve that vital B vitamin. For that reason, you need to serve it immediately.

serves 2
preparation time 5 minutes
cooking time 10 minutes

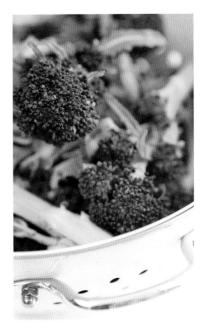

3¼ cups purple baby broccoli florets or other
   broccoli florets
1 tablespoon olive oil
2 cloves garlic, crushed
½ cup drained sun-dried tomatoes in oil
¼ cup slivered almonds, toasted

1 Steam the broccoli until just tender.
2 Meanwhile, heat the oil in a small saucepan and gently sauté the garlic until just soft, without browning.
3 Coarsely chop the tomatoes and stir into the garlicky oil.
4 When the broccoli is cooked, lift onto a serving plate and top with the tomato mixture. Sprinkle with the toasted almonds.

### serving suggestions
*This tastes great with broiled chicken thighs or plain fish.*

### allergens
*Nuts (almonds).*

# spinach with dried currants and pine nuts

Spinach is a great source of beta carotene, and your body converts it to vitamin A, which is particularly useful in the development of your baby's lungs. Here, the spinach is cooked Spanish style with pine nuts and dried currants, which enhance its nutritional credentials further with vitamin E and healthy monounsaturated fats. It should be served immediately (not stored) for the maximum retention of vitamins.

serves 2
preparation time 5 minutes
cooking time 10 minutes

2 tablespoons pine nuts
1 (10 oz) package fresh spinach leaves, well washed and drained
1 tablespoon olive oil
2 tablespoons dried currants
nutmeg

1 Toast the pine nuts in a dry skillet until they are lightly browned or in a preheated oven at 400°F. Be careful that they don't become overdone.
2 Meanwhile, put the drained spinach into a large saucepan and cook until it has completely wilted. You won't need additional water for this.
3 When the spinach has wilted, drain off the excess liquid and place in a serving dish.
4 Grate over some nutmeg, pour the olive oil over it, and stir in the dried currants and pine nuts. Serve hot immediately.

serving suggestions
*Delicious with any broiled or roasted meat, fish, or poultry, or stews.*

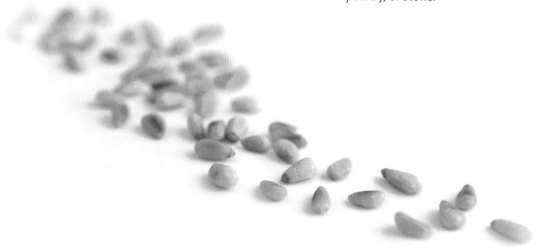

**COOK'S TIP**
*Not actually a nut but a seed of the pine tree, pine nuts are high in protein. While they can be eaten raw, toasting them brings out their buttery flavor and adds a little extra crunch.*

# roasted beet and butternut squash

Beet is rich in folate and butternut squash in beta-carotene, which your body turns to vitamin A. Both nutrients are pregnancy essentials and you and your baby will have at least one quarter of your day's needs in this easy, nutritious side dish.

serves 2
preparation time 10 minutes
cooking time 45 minutes

4 fresh beets
2 cups large butternut squash cubes
1 red onion, cut into wedges
2 tablespoons olive oil
chopped parsley, to garnish

1 Preheat the oven to 400°F.
2 Using plastic gloves to prevent your hands from staining, peel the beets and cut each into 8 wedges. Place in a roasting pan.
3 Add the squash and onion and drizzle with the olive oil. Give the pan a good shake or stir to coat the vegetables with the oil.
4 Roast for 40 to 45 minutes, until the vegetables are tender.
5 Serve sprinkled with a little parsley.

## serving suggestions
*Ideal with roasted or broiled meat, fish, or poultry. Try using any leftovers in* Barley and Roasted Vegetable Salad with Pumpkin Seeds, *page 71.*

## storage
*The roasted vegetables can be refrigerated for 24 hours and used in salads. They are not suitable for reheating or freezing.*

# spicy green edamame

Providing vitamin C as well as fiber, edamame (soybeans) are a welcome change to frozen peas. Here, they are stir-fried with green bell peppers, chile, and scallions for an Asian-style vegetable accompaniment.

serves 2
preparation time 5 minutes
cooking time 5 minutes

*2 teaspoons vegetable oil*
*½ large green bell pepper, sliced*
*3 scallions, trimmed and cut into ½ inch slices*
*1 green chile, finely chopped*
*⅔ cup edamame (soybeans), defrosted, if frozen*

1 Heat the oil in a nonstick wok or skillet.
2 Lightly sauté the bell pepper and scallions for 2 to 3 minutes before adding the chile, then the edamame.
3 Stir-fry for 3 to 4 minutes, or until the vegetables are just tender and piping hot. Serve immediately.

## serving suggestions
*Use to accompany* Chinese Pork with Plums *(page 97), tuna steaks, or any other hot dish of your choice.*

## allergens
*Soy (edamame).*

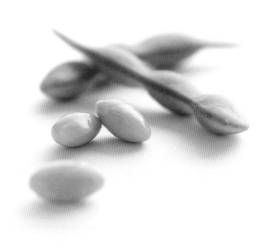

# almond rice

Adding a few slivered almonds to rice adds a nice crunch, but unfortunately won't add significant amounts of nutrients. However, almonds do provide antioxidant vitamin E, and a little calcium and iron, and this dish makes a change from plain boiled rice.

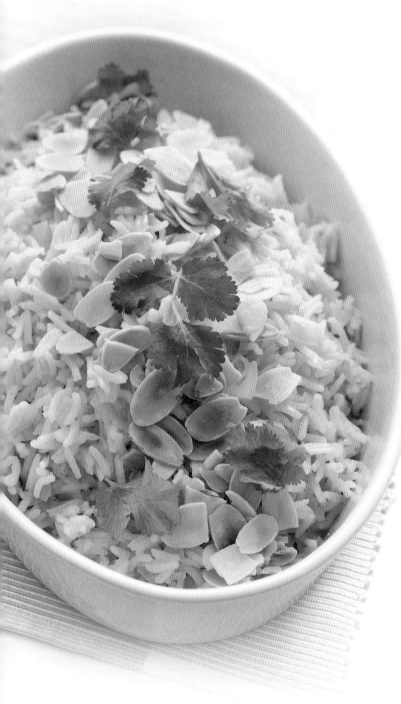

serves  2
preparation time  15 minutes
cooking time  15 minutes

*1 tablespoon vegetable oil*
*½ onion*
*½ cup basmati or other long grain rice, rinsed well*
  *and drained (see page 83)*
*1 cup boiling water*
*pinch of salt*
*1 bay leaf*
*⅓ cup slivered almonds, toasted*

**1** Add the oil to a saucepan and when hot, sauté the onion until lightly browned.
**2** Stir in the rinsed rice and water.
**3** Add the salt and bay leaf and bring to a boil.
**4** Cover the pan, lower the heat, and simmer for 10 minutes, or according to package directions, until all the water is absorbed.
**5** Remove the bay leaf and fluff up the rice with a fork.
**6** Sprinkle with the almonds before serving,

## serving suggestions
*Eat with* Tarka Dhal, *page 128, spicy stews, or curried dishes.*

## allergens
*Nuts (almonds).*

# orange and mint couscous

Store-bought flavored couscous is often high in sodium, but you can easily make your own salt-free tasty couscous that is cheaper, too. Choose the whole-grain version, if possible. This version uses a little boiling water to start the grains fluffing up, then unsweetened orange juice to provide vitamin C.

serves 2
preparation time 5 minutes
cooking time 0 minutes

*½ cup couscous, preferably whole grain*
*¼ cup boiling water*
*⅔ cup unsweetened orange juice*
*8 large mint leaves, finely chopped*

1 Put the couscous into a heatproof bowl, pour the boiling water over the grains, and let stand for 2 to 3 minutes.
2 Pour in the orange juice and let stand for an additional 5 or so minutes, or until all the juice has been absorbed.
3 Fork in the mint leaves and serve immediately.

## serving suggestions
*Use to accompany goulash, stews, or any meal where you may use rice. You may also add a spoonful of chopped seeds or nuts and a handful of dried fruit to make a delicious salad with any leftovers.*

## storage
*The couscous can be refrigerated for 24 hours, but is not suitable for freezing.*

## allergens
*Gluten (wheat).*

# herbed barley

Pearl barley is a great little grain, low on the glycemic index, full of fiber, and a great base for salads and soups as well as served as an alternative to rice, pasta, or potatoes. This recipe serves two, but if you make more, the remainder can be used for the delicious *Barley and Roasted Vegetable Salad with Pumpkin Seeds* on page 71.

serves 2
preparation time 5 minutes
cooking time 40 to 45 minutes

*½ cup pearl barley*
*1 cup low sodium vegetable broth*
*¼ cup finely chopped parsley*

1 Put the barley and broth into a small saucepan and bring to a boil.
2 Stir, cover, and reduce the temperature. Simmer gently for about 45 minutes, until all the broth has been absorbed and the grains are just tender.
3 Remove from the heat and stir in the chopped parsley and serve immediately.

## serving suggestions
*A great side dish for a casserole or goulash. Try using any leftovers in* Barley and Roasted Vegetable Salad with Pumpkin Seeds, *page 71.*

## storage
*The barley is best served soon after making, but can be kept in the refrigerator for 24 hours and used to make salads.*

## allergens
*Gluten (barley).*

# quinoa and sunflower seeds

Quinoa contains a lot of iron and zinc and is gluten free. It cooks fairly quickly and can make a delicious side dish to rival rice. It isn't rich in vitamins B or C, which are damaged from reheating, but it is an ideal grain to cook in bulk and freeze in individual portions to heat up later.

serves  2
preparation time  5 minutes
cooking time  15 to 20 minutes

¾ cup quinoa
1½ cups water
1 tablespoon sunflower seeds
2 teaspoons olive oil
black pepper
pinch of salt

1 Put the quinoa into a saucepan and pour the water over the grains. Bring to a boil, stir, and cover. Simmer gently, checking periodically, until all the water has been absorbed.
2 Meanwhile, toast the sunflower seeds either in a dry skillet on the stove or in a preheated oven, at 400°F, until just lightly browned and crisp.
3 When the quinoa is cooked, stir in the olive oil and season.
4 Put into a serving bowl and sprinkle with the seeds. Serve hot.

## serving suggestions
Good with roasted or broiled meat, fish, or poultry or stews.

## storage
The quinoa can be refrigerated for up to 48 hours, or frozen in small batches for up to 2 months. Defrost in the refrigerator and reheat in a microwave oven until piping hot.

# hot potato salad

My much healthier version of potato salad uses herbs and olive oil instead of mayonnaise and is served hot to retain vitamin C. The fresh herbs also add beneficial phytonutrients for you and your baby, as well as being a good replacement for salt.

serves  2
preparation time  5 minutes
cooking time  20 minutes

10 oz new potatoes, scrubbed clean and halved if large
2 tablespoons olive oil
3 scallions, cut into ½ inch slices
¼ cup mixed herbs such as parsley and mint, finely chopped

1 Steam or boil the potatoes until just tender, then drain.
2 While the potatoes are still hot, pour the olive oil them and toss with the herbs and scallions. Serve immediately.

## serving suggestions
Use to accompany roasted meat or poultry or broiled fish.

## storage
The salad can be cooled and refrigerated overnight but is best and most nutritious served hot.

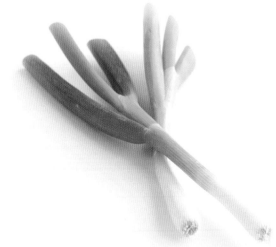

# gratin of potato

This is a good accompaniment to an oven cooked casserole, because it can bake alongside and be ready at the same time. Instead of the usual heavy cream, this is made with skim milk, keeping the fat content down and increasing the amount of calcium. One portion provides more than one quarter of your daily calcium requirement.

serves  2
preparation time  10 minutes
cooking time  1 to 1½ hours

3 white round or red-skinned potatoes
⅔ cup skim milk
pinch of salt
pinch grated nutmeg
¼ cup shredded cheddar cheese
few fresh rosemary sprigs, optional

1 Preheat the oven to 325°F. Oil a small ovenproof gratin dish.
2 Peel the potatoes and slice them as thinly as you can, using a mandoline slicer if you have one.
3 Rinse the potatoes well and pat dry on a clean dish towel.
4 Arrange the potato slices in layers in the dish.
5 Season the milk with salt, if using, black pepper, and nutmeg and pour the sauce over the potatoes.
6 Cover loosely with aluminum foil, place on a baking sheet in case of spillage, and place in the oven for about 1 hour.
7 Remove from the oven and pierce with a sharp knife to test if the potatoes are tender. Return for longer if not soft, or if now tender, sprinkle with the cheese and return to the oven, with rosemary sprigs, if using, but without the foil to crisp.

### COOK'S TIP
You can use new potatoes to make this gratin, which will increase the vitamin C content. Or if you want, add crushed garlic when layering the potatoes.

### serving suggestions
Use to accompany casseroles or stews, or broiled meat or poultry with sauce.

### storage
The gratin can be reheated although the vitamin content will be reduced. Refrigerate for up to 48 hours and reheat in a microwave oven until piping hot.

### allergens
Milk.

vegetables and side dishes

# DESSERTS AND BAKING

## orange and pomegranate salad

Very rich in vitamin C, this refreshing dessert works well in the winter months when both fruits are abundant. Oranges are also a great source of folate, which is needed early on.

serves 2
preparation time 10 minutes
cooking time 0 minutes

2 medium-large oranges
2/3 cup pomegranate seeds
2 tablespoons unsweetened orange juice, optional
1 tablespoon honey
2 or 3 mint leaves, finely chopped
seeds from 3 cardamon pods, ground, or pinch of
    ground cardamon
Greek-style yogurt (fat-free), to serve

1 Using a amall sharp knife, slice off the top and bottom of the orange. Set it on its bottom and cut off a strip of peel from top to bottom, removing the white pith. Continue all around the orange until it is completely pith free. Then lay on its side and cut into thin slices, reserving the juice.
2 Put the orange slices and pomegranate seeds into a serving dish.
3 Mix the honey with the reserved juice, or use store-bought juice if your oranges were not juicy. Stir in the mint and cardamom, then pour over the fruit.
4 Serve immediately, adding a dollop of yogurt, or cover with plastic wrap and chill until required.

### storage
*Best served immediately, but will keep in the refrigerator for 24 hours, with some vitamin C and folic acid loss.*

## raspberry and pomegranate gelatin

Raspberries are a wonderful source of vitamin C as well as flavones and phenols, which boost your immune system. Moms-to-be who have pregnancy diabetes can use the natural sweetener, xylitol.

serves 4
preparation time 15 minutes
cooking time 0 minutes

1 (1/4 oz) envelope plain gelatin powder
2 1/2 tablespoons superfine sugar or xylitol
1/4 cup red fruit cordial, such as grenadine or cassis
    or sugar-free fruit syrup
1 cup fresh raspberries
1 cup pomegranate seeds

1 Make the gelatin by pouring 1/4 cup of hot, but not boiling water into a small heatproof bowl, and sprinkle the gelatin over it. Let stand for a couple of minutes, then stir to dissolve the gelatin.
2 Dissolve the sugar or xylitol in 1/2 cup cold water and add to the bowl of dissolved gelatin.
3 Add the cordial or syrup and enough water to make up 2 cups of gelatin.
4 Put the raspberries and pomegranate seeds into a serving dish. Pour the gelatin mixture over them and refrigerate to set for at least a couple of hours.

### serving suggestions
*Accompany with vanilla ice cream, or a spoonful of lowfat Greek yogurt.*

### storage
*The gelatin can be refrigerated for 2 to 3 days. It is not suitable for freezing.*

# strawberry mousse

Homemade mousses and souffles are usually off limits in pregnancy, because they use raw egg white. However, if you use dried egg white powder, which is pasteurized, you can enjoy light desserts without worry. Here, dried egg white is used to make a meringue into which you simply fold strawberry puree and fromage frais. When strawberries are at their peak, this low-fat, vitamin C-rich dish will go down easily.

serves  4
preparation time  10 minutes
cooking time  0 minutes

4 teaspoons egg white powder
¼ cup warm water
¼ cup superfine sugar
1 lb strawberries, hulled, and halved; reserve a few
   for decoration
1¼ cup fromage frais, quark or Greek-style yogurt

## FOOD SAFETY
*Do not use raw egg white for this recipe.*

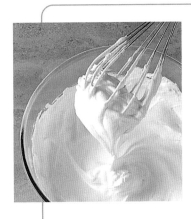

### MAKING MERINGUE
*To check that your egg whites are the right consistency, lift your whisk. The mixture below should stand up without curling over.*

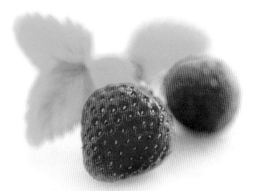

1 Put the egg white powder into a large mixing bowl and stir in 2 tablespoons of the warm water. Mix well to dissolve, pour in the remaining water, and whisk until the egg white is light and forms peaks.
2 Add the sugar and continue whisking until you have a thick glossy meringue.
3 Puree the strawberries in a blender, and carefully fold into the meringue.
4 Fold in the fromage frais and then pour the mousse into 4 individual serving dishes.
5 Chill until required, then serve topped with the reserved strawberries.

### serving suggestions
*You can eat it with a plain sweet cookie.*

### storage
*The mousse can be kept covered in plastic wrap in the refrigerator for 2 days. It is not suitable for freezing.*

### allergens
*Eggs.*

desserts and baking

# dried fruit salad

Great for a simple dessert, this dish is rich in fiber and one serving provides about 20 percent of your day's need for iron. Choose different dried fruits but keep in mind that figs, apricots, and raisins are higher in iron than prunes, pears, or apples, and figs are best for calcium. It also makes a terrific breakfast.

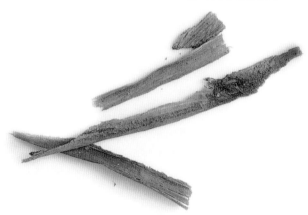

serves 3
preparation time 5 minutes
chilling time overnight

9 dried figs, halved if large, and stalk removed
9 dried prunes
3 tablespoons raisins
9 dried apricot halves
1½ dried apple rings
1 cup unsweetened orange juice
1 cinnamon stick or vanilla bean, or both (optional)
plain yogurt, to serve

1 Put all the fruit into a bowl and pour the juice over them.
2 Add the cinnamon or vanilla, if using.
3 Cover with plastic wrap and refrigerate overnight.
4 Remove the cinnamon stick and/or vanilla bean before serving and top with a dollop of yogurt.

## storage
*This salad will keep in the refrigerator for 2 to 3 days.*

# summer fruit compote

Rich in vitamin C and protective polyphenols, this compote is an easy way to have two of your five a day in one easy dish.

serves 2
preparation time 5 minutes
cooking time 5 minutes

2½ cups frozen mixed berries, thawed or
  1 cup blackberries
¾ cup blueberries or black currants
¾ cup raspberries
¼ cup superfine sugar or xylitol

1 If using frozen fruit, place the defrosted fruit in a small saucepan and add the sugar or xylitol.
2 Bring gradually to simmering point, stir to dissolve the sugar, and then remove from the heat.
3 If using fresh fruit, put all the fruit except the raspberries into a saucepan with the sugar or xylitol. Bring to simmering point, then stir in the raspberries. Remove from the heat.
4 Let cool and serve at room temperature, or if you prefer, chill.

## serving suggestions
*Eat with a spoonful of Greek yogurt.*

## storage
*The compote can be refrigerated in an airtight container for 2 to 3 days. It can also be frozen for up to 3 months.*

> **COOK'S TIP**
> *Make a simple fruit coulis by blending the fruit compote and storing it in several freezer bags in the freezer for up to 3 months.*

# mango and lime dessert

Mangoes are an amazing source of vitamins A and C, which are essential for your baby's eye development, as well as keeping you healthy during pregnancy. This dessert uses calcium-rich tofu, which makes this dessert ideal if you can't tolerate dairy foods..

serves  2
preparation time  10 minutes
cooking time  0 minutes

*1 ripe mango or 2 cups mango cubes*
*6 oz silken tofu*
*grated zest of 1 lime*
*1 tablespoon lime juice*
*½ teaspoon vanilla extract*

1 If using a whole mango, peel and cut into cubes.
2 Put all the ingredients into a food processor or blender and process until smooth.
3 Spoon into 2 serving dishes, and chill until required.

## serving suggestions
*Accompany with a sweet plain cookie.*

## storage
*This dessert can be refrigerated, covered with plastic wrap for a day or two. It is not suitable for freezing.*

## allergens
*Soy.*

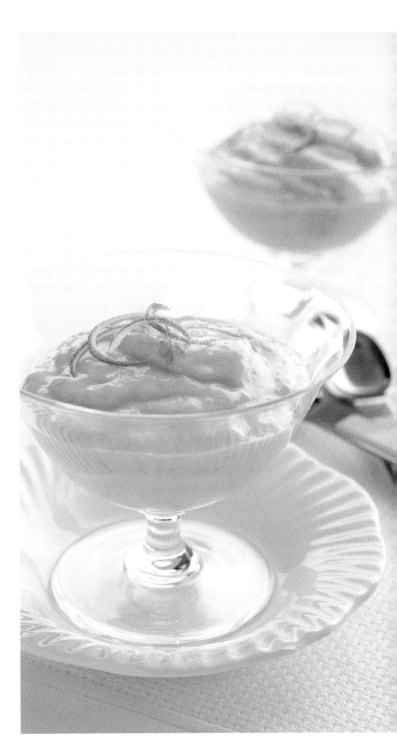

### DICING A MANGO
*Slice the flesh of the two pitless sections in a lattice pattern, cutting down to the peel but not piercing it. Push the peel inside out with your thumbs. Cut away cubes with a knife.*

# pears in chocolate sauce

Pears are easily digested and a good source of fiber. They are served here with a chocolate sauce, but if you want a lower fat option, choose a store-bought fruity coulis, or make your own by blending a little of the Summer Fruit Compote (page 142).

serves 2
preparation time 15 minutes
cooking time 45 minutes

2 large ripe pears that will stand upright in a
    saucepan (such as Comice)
1¼ cups grape juice
1 vanilla bean

for the chocolate sauce
*(makes enough for 3 servings)*
*2 oz dark chocolate with at least 70% cocoa solids*
*1 tablespoon butter*
*1 tablespoon packed light brown sugar*
*¼ cup reduced fat light cream*

1 Peel the pears carefully, leaving the stem, if present. It can be useful for maneuvering the pear later.
2 Stand the pears upright in a small saucepan and add the grape juice and vanilla bean. Cover and cook over gentle heat for 40 to 45 minutes, occasionally spooning some of the cooking liquid over the pears.
3 When the pears are tender, remove from the heat and carefully lift into a serving bowl. Discard or reuse the vanilla bean and let the cooking liquid cool to serve with the pears.
4 Meanwhile, while the pears are poaching, melt the chocolate and butter in a small heatproof bowl over a saucepan of just simmering water.
6 When they are melted, stir in the sugar until it dissolves, then add the cream.
7 Stir and pour into a small pitcher.
8 Serve the poached pears with their juice and some chocolate sauce poured over them.

## storage
*The pears, once cooked, can be stored in an airtight container and refrigerated for up to 2 days. The sauce may also be refrigerated. Neither are suitable for freezing.*

## allergens
*Milk (butter and cream).*

# traditional rice pudding

This easy-to-prepare pudding is ideal for days when you may feel a little nauseous, and a single serving contains nearly half of your day's needs for calcium.

serves  4
preparation time  5 minutes
cooking time  1½ to 2 hours

*3 cups lowfat milk*
*⅓ cup short grain rice.*
*¼ cup superfine sugar or xylitol*
*2–3 strips of lemon zest*
*whole nutmeg for grating*

1 Preheat the oven to 300°F.
2 Oil a 1 quart ovenproof dish.
3 Mix the rice, milk, and sugar or xylitol in the dish, and add the strips of lemon zest.
4 Cover the surface with finely grated nutmeg and bake for 1½ to 2 hours, or until the pudding has a caramel colored brown crust and the rice is tender and soft.
5 Serve immediately, removing the lemon zest when you find them.

## serving suggestions
*Accompany with Summer Fruit Compote or Dried Fruit Salad (both on page 142).*

## storage
*The pudding can be covered with plastic wrap and refrigerated for up to 2 days. Reheat in a microwave oven to prevent it from drying out. It is not suitable for freezing.*

## allergens
*Milk.*

# honey-roasted stone fruit

Summer time brings a host of succulent "stone" fruit (fruit with pits). Enjoy a selection roasted with honey for a boost of vitamin C and an easily digested dessert.

serves  2
preparation time  5 minutes
cooking time  15 to 20 minutes

*1 ripe peach or nectarine*
*2 ripe apricots*
*2 ripe plums*
*8 cherries, pitted*
*2 tablespoons honey*

1 Preheat the oven to 350°F.
2 Wash the fruit and cut the larger fruits in half. Remove the pits, and cut in half again.
3 Put all the fruit into a small ovenproof dish and drizzle with the honey
4 Bake for 15 to 20 minutes, or until the fruit is just tender.
5 Serve immediately with any cooking juices.

## serving suggestions
Top with a dollop of low-fat Greek yogurt.

## storage
*The fruit can be stored in an airtight container and refrigerated for up to 2 days. It is not suitable for freezing.*

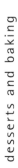

desserts and baking

# baked figs with pistachios and honey yogurt

Fresh figs are a wonderful source of fiber and make a delicious, inexpensive hot dessert when they are in season. There are several varieties of figs available in smaller and larger sizes from late summer into fall. Choose fruit that are plump and tender but not soft. Figs that are not ripe can be ripened by placing them on a sunny windowsill for a day or two.

serves  2
preparation time  10 minutes
cooking time  15 to 20 minutes

1 or 2 figs per person
2 tablespoons honey
2/3 cup Greek-style plain yogurt
2 tablespoons coarsely chopped unsalted
  pistachio nuts

1 Preheat the oven to 375°F.
2 Wash the figs and cut in half from vertically, from stem to the bottom.
3 Put the figs into a small ovenproof dish and spoon the honey over them. Bake, uncovered, for 15 to 20 minutes, until the figs are soft and heated through.
4 Remove from the oven and place the figs in 2 serving dishes, saving the honeyed cooking juices.
5 Put the yogurt into a small mixing bowl and stir in the cooking juices. Spoon half next to the figs and sprinkle with the pistachios. Serve immediately.

## storage
*The cooked figs can be stored in the refrigerator. Make the honeyed yogurt and store separately, but don't add the nuts until serving. Not suitable for freezing.*

## allergens
*Milk (yogurt), nuts (pistachio).*

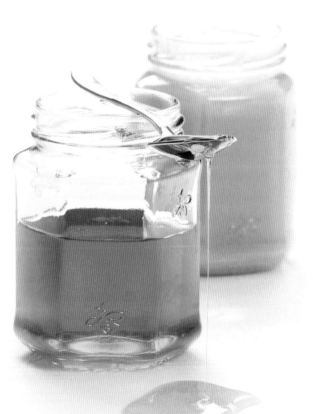

### COOK'S TIP
*To measure the honey accurately, dip the spoon into a cup of hot water before measuring.*

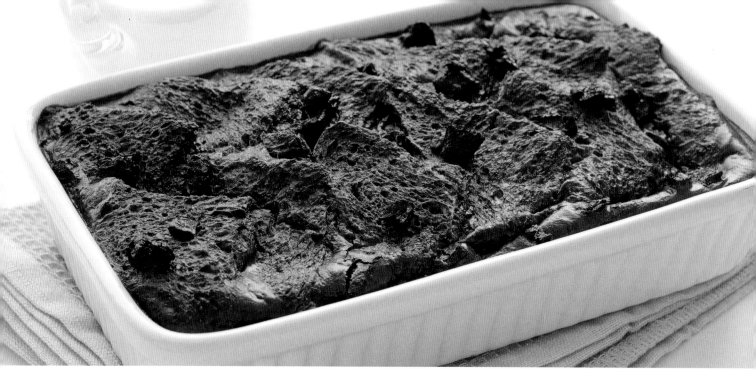

# chocolate brioche pudding

A comforting and fluffy bread and butter pudding made with sweet brioche bread and a sweet chocolate egg custard. Adding a few prunes increases sweetness (and fiber content) without the need for much additional sugar.

serves  3
preparation time  10 minutes
cooking time  30 to 35 minutes

*¼ cup unsweetened cocoa powder*
*1 tablespoon sugar*
*1 cup lowfat milk*
*2 eggs, beaten*
*1 teaspoon vanilla extract*
*3½ oz sliced brioche loaf*
*6 pitted prunes, coarsely chopped*

1 Preheat the oven to 350°F.
2 Grease a 1 quart ovenproof dish
3 Mix the cocoa powder and sugar with a little of the milk until smooth. Add the remaining milk, eggs, and vanilla to make a custard mixture.
4 Cut the slices of bread diagonally in half or quarters, depending on the size of your dish. Place a layer in the bottom of the dish, add half the prunes, and pour half of the chocolate mixture over the top. Repeat.
5 Bake until the pudding is light and fluffy and when you insert a knife, the egg custard is no longer runny.

### serving suggestions
*Top with a spoonful of reduced fat light cream.*

### storage
*The pudding can be kept covered in the refrigerator for 2 to 3 days, and if reheated must be piping hot.*

### allergens
*Gluten (wheat), eggs, milk.*

#### COOK'S TIP
*A good quality bread, such as brioche (which is egg-rich), gives the best results.*

desserts and baking

# apple and berry oat crisp

This simple dessert uses fresh apples and a can of berries in juice. Whether you use fresh, frozen, or canned berries, they all contain nutrients. Using canned fruit in juice means you don't need to sweeten the apples with sugar. If you use frozen or fresh, add unsweetened apple juice.

serves  4
preparation time  10 minutes
cooking time  25 to 30 minutes

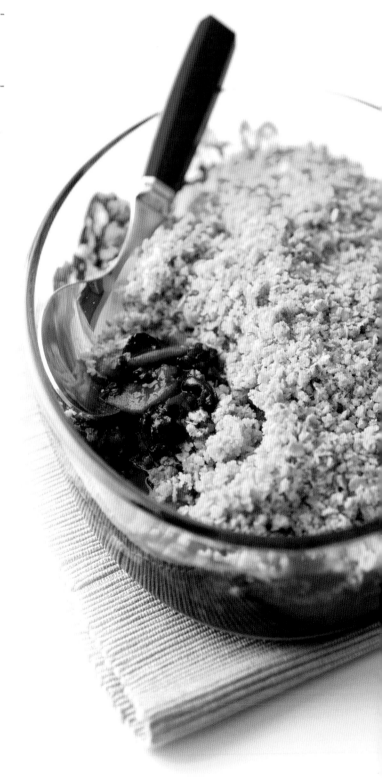

2 cooking apples, such as Granny Smiths, peeled
10 oz canned black currants, blueberries, or cherries
  in juice
1 teaspoon cornstarch
2/3 cup all-purpose flour
1/4 cup packed light brown sugar
1 cup rolled oats
pinch of cinnamon
1/4 cup polyunsaturated spread (not fat reduced)

1 Preheat the oven to 375°F. Grease a 1½ quart ovenproof dish

2 Slice the apples into thin slices. Drain the berries, reserving the juice, and put into the dish. Stir the cornstarch into the berry juice, then pour it over the fruit.

3 Sift the flour into a mixing bowl, and add the sugar, oats, and cinnamon. Rub in the spread until the mixture is all combined.

4 Spoon the crisp topping over the fruit and bake for 25 to 30 minutes, or until the crisp is golden brown and the apples are tender when you insert a knife. Serve immediately.

## serving suggestions
*Accompany with custard, some lowfat quark or yogurt, or vanilla ice cream.*

## storage
*The crisp is best served on the day it is made but can be kept in the refrigerator for 2 days. It can also be frozen for up to 2 months.*

## allergens
*Gluten (oats, wheat).*

# fruity oat bars

Add zinc to your pregnancy diet in a palatable way with these oat bars made with pumpkin seeds and figs, both of which are a great source of this essential mineral. One slice will provide you with 15 percent of your day's need for zinc and 10 percent of iron.

serves  16
preparation time  15 minutes
cooking time  30 to 35 minutes

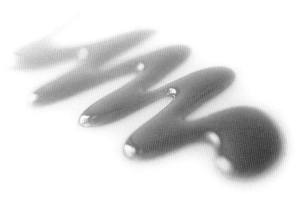

¾ cup sunflower spread (not reduced fat)
⅓ cup maple syrup
¼ cup packed light brown sugar
½ cup chopped dried dates
2 figs, chopped
⅔ cup chopped dried apricots
½ cup pumpkin seeds
2¾ cups rolled oats (see tip)

1  Preheat the oven to 375°F.
2  Grease a 10 inch square baking pan.
3  Heat the sunflower spread, syrup, and sugar in a saucepan over low heat until they are melted, stirring occasionally. Be careful to avoid boiling the mixture.
4  Stir in the chopped dates and continue to heat gently for a minute or two to soften the dates.
5  Meanwhile, combine all the remaining dry ingredients in a large mixing bowl.
6  Pour the date syrup mixture into the bowl and stir until all the dry ingredients are coated with the syrup.
7  Spoon into the prepared pan and level the mixture by pressing down with the back of a clean spoon.

8  Bake until the mixture just turns golden, then remove from the oven and let cool for a few minutes.
9  Before the mixture sets completely, cut into 16 pieces with a sharp knife, then let cool in the pan.
10 When cold, carefully remove the oat bars and store in an airtight container until required.

## serving suggestions
*Eat with a glass of milk or juice.*

## storage
*The oat bars keep well for up to a week in an airtight container in a cool dry place. They may be frozen for up to 3 months.*

## allergens
*Gluten (oats).*

### COOK'S TIP
*When making flapjacks with lots of extra ingredients you may find the mixture holds together better if you use the less expensive rolled oats as well as or instead of jumbo oats.*

desserts and baking

# carrot sheet cake

While one could not claim that eating cake is a pregnancy essential, this cake does at least provide one third of your day's needs of vitamin A, thanks to the carrots it contains. Make one to freeze for when your baby is born and you have plenty of admiring visitors—but it won't just be the baby they'll be praising.

serves  16
preparation time  15 minutes
cooking time  35 to 40 minutes

1 cup vegetable (canola) oil
¾ cup firmly packed light brown sugar
3 eggs
1½ cups finely shredded carrot
¾ cup whole wheat flour
¾ cup white all-purpose flour
3 teaspoon baking powder
1 teaspoon ground cinnamon
½ cup coarsely chopped walnuts

for the frosting
2 tablespoons unsalted butter
3 tablespoons cream cheese or mascarpone
1 tablespoon lemon juice
1¼ cups confectioners' sugar, sifted

1 Preheat the oven to 350°F.
2 Line a 10 inch square baking pan with parchment paper and oil lightly.
3 Pour the oil into a large bowl, then beat in the sugar and eggs until the mixture is paler and the volume has increased.
4 Fold in the carrots.
5 Sift the flours, baking powder, and cinnamon together and fold into the mixture, adding any bran that has remained in the sifter.
6 Fold in the walnuts and transfer the batter into the prepared pan.
7 Bake for 35 to 40 minutes, or until the cake springs back when lightly pressed.
8 Cool on a wire rack while making the topping.

for the frosting and assembly
1 Beat together the butter and cream cheese or mascarpone and gradually stir in the confectioners' sugar and a teaspoon of the lemon juice.
2 If the mixture is still stiff, add a little more lemon juice and beat well until the frosting is smooth.
3 Use a spatula to spread the frosting over the cooled cake, and use a fork to create a decorative pattern on the top.
4 Chill until required.

serving suggestions
Great as an afternoon snack or as a dessert after a light lunch or dinner.

storage
The cake can be refrigerated for 3 to 4 days, or frozen for up to 3 months. Defrost in the refrigerator.

allergens
Gluten (wheat), eggs, milk (butter/cream cheese), nuts (walnuts).

> **NUTRITION NOTE**
> *Choosing canola oil as the vegetable oil will make this sponge cake low in saturates and high in monounsaturates, so you can use butter and cream cheese in the frosting without worrying you will have an overly rich cake.*

# orange bran muffins

Whether for breakfast or a snack with a glass of milk or cup of herb tea, these easy-to-make muffins supply you with essential fiber, as well a small amount of iron and vitamin C. Make a batch and freeze—they defrost quickly so you can enjoy one at any time, even when you have a fit of the midnight munchies.

serves 12
preparation time 10 minutes
cooking time 20 minutes

1²/₃ cups All Bran
1¼ cups unsweetened orange juice
²/₃ cup raisins
2 eggs
¼ cup granulated sugar
¼ cup vegetable oil
2 cups all-purpose flour
1 tablespoon baking powder

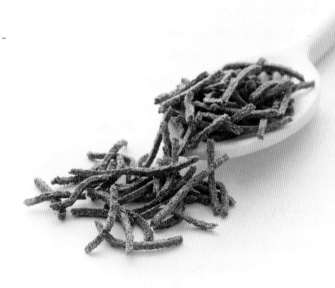

1 Preheat the oven to 375°F.
2 Put 12 paper muffin liners into a muffin pan.
3 Soak the All Bran and raisins in the orange juice for 5 minutes while you prepare the remaining ingredients.
4 Whisk the eggs in a large bowl with the sugar and oil until combined.
5 Sift the flour and baking powder together.
6 Pour the bran mixture into the egg mixture and beat well.
7 Fold in the flour to make a thick batter.
8 Spoon the batter into the muffin liners and bake for 20 minutes, or until the tops are springy to the touch.
9 Cool and serve as required.

### serving suggestions
*Eat with fresh sliced oranges and plain yogurt for a simple breakfast or with a glass of milk for a nourishing midmorning snack.*

### storage
*The muffins can be kept for 2 days in an airtight container, or frozen for up to 3 months.*

### allergens
*Gluten (wheat), eggs.*

# chocolate brazil brownies

Brazil nuts are one of the few good sources of the antioxidant selenium, which help protect you and your baby. If you are chocolate addict, eat one of these instead of a chocolate bar, because they will provide you and your baby with more nutrients.

serves  12
preparation time  15 minutes
cooking time  30 to 35 minutes

2½ oz dark chocolate (at least 70% cocoa solids)
⅓ cup sunflower spread (not reduced fat)
2 eggs, beaten
¾ cup packed light brown sugar
1 teaspoon vanilla extract
¾ cup all-purpose flour
¾ teaspoon baking powder
½ cup coarsely chopped Brazil nuts

### for the frosting
2 oz dark chocolate (at least 70% cocoa solids)
⅔ cup confectioners' sugar, sifted
1 tablespoon water
½ teaspoon vanilla extract
8 Brazil nuts, chopped

1 Preheat the oven to 350°F.
2 Line an 8 inch square baking pan with parchment paper and oil lightly.
3 Put the chocolate and sunflower spread into a heatproof bowl and melt over a saucepan of barely simmering water.
4 When melted, remove the bowl and beat in the eggs, sugar, and vanilla.
5 Stir in the flour, baking powder, and nuts, and pour the batter into the prepared pan.
6 Bake for 30 to 35 minutes or until the brownies are just springy to the touch. Cool.
7 To make the frosting, melt the chocolate in a small heatproof bowl over a saucepan of barely simmering water.
8 Stir in the confectioners' sugar, vanilla extract, and just enough water to make a thick but spreadable frosting.

9 Using a spactual, spread the frosting over the brownies, sprinkle with the Brazil nuts, and let set before cutting into 12 pieces.

### serving suggestions
*Delicious with a cup of tea, or have as a dessert with a scoop of vanilla ice cream.*

### storage
*The brownies can be frozen for up to 3 months in an airtight container, or stored for a few days in a cool dry cupboard.*

### allergens
*Wheat (gluten), eggs, nuts (Brazils).*

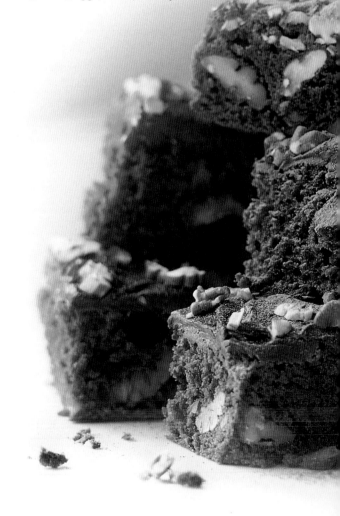

# Cheddar and sun-dried tomato biscuits

Biscuits make a welcome change to sandwiches or bread with a soup lunch. One of these biscuits provides one quarter of your day's calcium needs.

serves 8
preparation time 10 minutes
cooking time 15 minutes

1¼ cups white all-purpose flour
¾ cup whole wheat flour
1 tablespoon baking powder
½ cup drained and coarsely chopped sun-dried tomatoes in oil
1 cup shredded reduced fat cheddar cheese
1¼ cups buttermilk
a little milk as required

1   Preheat the oven to 450°F. Grease a baking sheet.
2   Sift the 2 flours and baking powder into a mixing bowl, adding any bran that remains in the sifter.
3   Add the tomatoes and ¾ cup of the cheese.
4   Stir in the buttermilk to make a soft but not sticky dough. Add a little milk if it is too dry, or more flour if too sticky.

5   Put the baking sheet into the oven to heat up while you prepare the dough.
6   Place the dough on a floury surface and lightly roll out to about ¾ inch in thickness. Using a round cutter, cut out 8 biscuits.
7   Remove the hot baking sheet from the oven and place the biscuits on it.
8   Brush the top of each scone with a little milk and sprinkle with the remaining cheese.
9   Bake for 12 to 15 minutes, or until the biscuits are just golden brown.
10  Cool slightly and serve.

### serving suggestions
*Spread with lowfat cream cheese and eat with a piece of celery or use to accompany a bowl of soup.*

### storage
*The biscuits are best on the day they are made, but can be frozen for up to 3 months. They will quickly defrost and can be reheated successfully in a microwave oven.*

### allergens
*Gluten (wheat), milk (buttermilk and cheese).*

<chocolate Brazil brownies

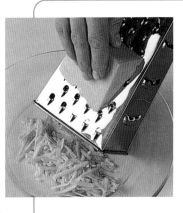

### SHREDDING CHEESE
*An upright grater is quick and easy to use, making coarse shreds. A rotary grater may be better if you want the cheese to be finer. For the best results, shred cheese straight from the refrigerator.*

# NUTRITIONAL ANALYSIS

Each recipe has been analyzed on a single serving amount. Where a recipe has a useful amount of the recommended daily intake of micronutrients during pregnancy, these amounts have also been included.

**Almond rice:** Energy 349 cal; Protein 7.8g; Carbohydrate 43.5g of which sugars 2.1g; Fat 15.8g of which saturates 1.2g; Fiber 2.7g; Sodium 200mg.

**Apple and berry oat crisp:** Energy 300 cal; Protein 4.6g; Carbohydrate 52.2g of which sugars 26.5g; Fat 10.5g of which saturates 2.3g; Fiber 7.3g; Sodium 100mg; Iron 5.1mg; Vitamin C 19.5mg.

**Apple, sage, and walnut sauce:** Energy 90 cal; Protein 1.5g; Carbohydrate 7.8g of which sugars 7.7g; Fat 6.1g of which saturates 0.5g; Fiber 1.5g; Sodium 0mg.

**Asparagus risotto:** (analyzed with water and vermouth not broth). Energy 477 cal; Protein 16.0g; Carbohydrate 61.1g of which sugars 5.7g; Fat 16.8g of which saturates 4.4g; Fiber 5.3g; Sodium 200mg; Calcium 212mg.

**Baba ganoush with bread and asparagus tips:** Energy 293 cal; Protein 12.1g; Carbohydrate 32.5g of which sugars 4.8g; Fat 13g of which saturates 3.7g; Fiber 11.2g; Calcium 245mg; Iron 3.85mg; Zinc 2.35mg; Folate 96mcg.

**Baked beef and sour cherries:** Energy 374 cal; Protein 30.4g; Carbohydrate 40.7g of which sugars 12.7g; Fat 7.3g of which saturates 1.9g; Fiber 2.2g; Sodium 80mg; Iron 3.72mg; Zinc 7.34mg; Vitamin A 274mcg; Vitamin $B_3$ (niacin) 3.4mg; Vitamin $B_6$ 0.41mg; Vitamin $B_{12}$ 2.5mcg.

**Baked figs with pistachios and honey yogurt:** Energy 206 cal; Protein 7.4g; Carbohydrate 26.65g of which sugars 26.2g; Fat 8.6g of which saturates 2.2g; Fiber 3.8g; Sodium 80mg; Calcium 195mg.

**Barley and roasted vegetable salad with pumpkin seeds:** Energy 480 cal; Protein 20.1g; Carbohydrate 64.4g of which sugars 14.5g; Fat 20.1g of which saturates 3.0g; Fiber 13.1g; Sodium 240mg; Vitamin C 30mg; Folate 80mcg; Vitamin A 560mcg; Iron 6.3mg; Magnesium 143mg.

**Bean and salsa wrap:** Energy 345 cal; Protein 19.2g; Carbohydrate 52.4g of which sugars 4.5g; Fat 5.8g of which saturates 2.5g; Fiber 7.6g; Sodium 800mg; Calcium 360mg; Vitamin A 350mcg.

**Beef and beet sandwich:** Energy 450 cal; Protein 29.7g; Carbohydrate 44.0g of which sugars 8.3g; Fat 18.6g of which saturates 5.1g; Fiber 7.9g; Sodium 720mg; Iron 4.5mg; Zinc 6.0mg; Folate 92mcg.

**Beef in beer:** Energy 323 cal; Protein 28.0g; Carbohydrate 20.3g of which sugars 12.1g; Fat 12.7g of which saturates 3.2g; Fiber 4.9g; Sodium 160mg; Zinc 7.3mg; Copper 0.43mg; Vitamin A 1,560mcg.

**Berry yogurt breakfast:** Energy 226 cal; Protein 12.5g; Carbohydrate 26.8g of which sugars 23.6g; Fat 8.4g of which saturates 1.0g; Fiber 6.3g; Sodium100mg; Calcium 280mg; Vitamin C 55mg; Zinc 2.0mg; Vitamin E 6.0mg.

**Blackberry sauce:** Energy 60 cal; Protein 0.5 g; Carbohydrate 10.6g of which sugars 10.6g; Fat 0.1g of which saturates 0g; Fiber 2.7g; Sodium 0g.

*Black*-eyed pea, dried currant, and fresh mint stew: Energy 276 cal; Protein 12.9g; Carbohydrate 44.4g of which sugars 19.7g; Fat 7.1g of which saturates 1.0g; Fiber 6.1g; Sodium trace; Folate 137mcg; Vitamin $B_1$ (thiamin) 0.24mg; Iron 5.4mg; Phosphorus 232mg.

**Brazil nut burgers:** Energy 406 cal; Protein 10.5g; Carbohydrate 42.3g of which sugars 11.6g; Fat 22.8g of which saturates 5.0g; Fiber 3.9g; Sodium 520mg; Calcium 175mg; Selenium 69mcg.

**Broccoli with almonds:** Energy 228 cal; Protein 8.3 g; Carbohydrate 4.5 g of which sugars 3.0 g; Fat 19.8 g of which saturates 1.6 g; Fiber 4.9g; Sodium 0g; Calcium 260mg; Vitamin C 63mg; Folate 110 mcg.

**Butternut squash casserole with halloumi and pomegranate:** Energy 461 cal; Protein 18.4g; Carbohydrate 55.3g of which sugars 26.7g; Fat 20.1g of which saturates 9g; Fiber 9.6g; Sodium 600mg; Magnesium 99mg; Folate 75mcg; Vitamin C 40mg; Vitamin A 2,030 mcg.

**Carrot sheet cake** ($^1/_{16}$ cake including frosting). Energy 285 cal; Protein 3.3g; Carbohydrate 29.1g of which sugars 20.1g; Fat 18.4g of which saturates 3.0g; Fiber 1.6g; Sodium 0g; Vitamin A 230mcg; Vitamin E 3.2mg.

**Casserole of duck and shallots with peaches:** Energy 178 cal; Protein 14.3g; Carbohydrate 8.9g of which sugars 8.9g; Fat 9.8g of which saturates 1.7g; Fiber 3.4g; Sodium 100mg; Zinc 2.62 mg; Copper 0.3 mg.

**Cheddar and sun-dried tomato biscuits:** Energy 175 cal; Protein 8.9g; Carbohydrate 24.6g of which sugars 2.1g; Fat 5.0g of which saturates 1.4g; Fiber 2.3g; Sodium 100mg; Calcium 75mg.

**Chinese beef and noodles:** Energy 474 cal; Protein 30.6g; Carbohydrate 67.2g of which sugars 4.6g; Fat 11.1g of which saturates 2.2g; Fiber 7.4g; Sodium 1,080mg; Iron 5.0mg; Zinc 4.6mg; Vitamin $B_3$ (niacin) 7.0mg; Vitamin $B_1$ (thiamin) 0.23mg.

**Chinese pork with plums:** Energy 374 cal; Protein 35.3g; Carbohydrate 33.8g of which sugars 30.8g; Fat 12.0g of which saturates 2.5g; Fiber 5.1g; Sodium 80mg; Vitamin $B_1$ (thiamin) 1.0mg; Vitamin $B_6$ 0.67mg; Zinc 3.6mg.

**Chicken with pine nuts and prunes:** Energy 366 cal; Protein 30g; Carbohydrate 25.1g of which sugars 24.2g; Fat 15.2g of which saturates 1.8g; Fiber 5.8g; Sodium 120mg; Iron 3.85mg; Potassium 1,165mg; Vitamin E 2.7mg.

**Chocolate and spicy chicken:** (analyzed without yogurt). Energy 265 cal; Protein 23.1g; Carbohydrate 23.6g of which sugars 22.4g; Fat 7.5g of which saturates 1.6g; Fiber 3.3g; Sodium 160mg; Potassium 915mg; Zinc 2.3mg; Copper 0.36 mg.

**Chocolate Brazil brownies:** Energy 261 cal; Protein 3.7g; Carbohydrate 32.7g of which sugars 26.4g; Fat 14.1g of which saturates 4.5g; Fiber 1.2g; Sodium 80mg; Selenium 23mcg.

**Chocolate brioche pudding:** Energy 280 cal; Protein 12.2g; Carbohydrate 36.2g of which sugars 20.6g; Fat 10.9g of which saturates 5.3g; Fiber 4.5g; Sodium 80mg; Vitamin $B_{12}$ 1.3 mcg.

**Chorizo and black-eyed peas with Israeli couscous:** (folate data based on boiled dried beans). Energy 380 cal; Protein 24.1g; Carbohydrate 44.9g of which sugars 5.5g; Fat 14.0g of which saturates 5. g; Fiber 11.4g; Sodium 160mg; Folate 150mcg; Vitamin A 700mcg.

**Citrus salad bowl:** Energy 70 cal; Protein 1.7g; Carbohydrate 16g of which sugars 15.8g; Fat 0.4g of which saturates 0g; Fiber 3.6g; Sodium 0g; Vitamin C 80mg.

nutritional analysis

**Crab cakes with watercress and orange salad:** Energy 484 cal; Protein 18.6g; Carbohydrate 32.6g of which sugars 12.8g; Fat 31.7g of which saturates 3.9g; Fiber 6.5g; Sodium 400mg; Calcium 175mg; Vitamin C 80mg; Iodine 120mcg; Omega 3 2.45g.

**Crab linguine:** Energy 514 cal; Protein 26.8g; Carbohydrate 58.8g of which sugars 4.7g; Fat 17.1g of which saturates 2.3g; Fiber 5.1g; Sodium 120mg; Magnesium 104 mg; Iron 4.5mg; Folic acid 90mcg; Omega 3 1.83g; Iodine 164mcg.

**Creamy vegetarian ground "beef":** Energy 236 cal; Protein 16.8g; Carbohydrate 8.8g of which sugars 6.4g; Fat 15.4g of which saturates 2.6g; Fiber 7.8g; Sodium 360mg; Zinc 6.1mg; Vitamin C 16.0mg; Copper 0.3mg.

**Curly kale with garlic cherry tomatoes:** Energy 85 cal; Protein 2.9 g; Carbohydrate 3.6g of which sugars 3.1g; Fat 6. g of which saturates 1.0g; Fiber 2.1g; Sodium trace; Vitamin A 374mcg; Vitamin C 43mg.

**Dried fruit salad:** Energy 187 cal; Protein 3.1g; Carbohydrate 44.8g of which sugars 44.8g; Fat 0.8g of which saturates 0g; Fiber 7.4g; Sodium 0g; Potassium 1,020mg; Vitamin C 26.4mg.

**Duck and Asian mushroom stir fry:** Energy 295 cal; Protein 25.5g; Carbohydrate 15.7g of which sugars 7.4g; Fat 13.5g of which saturates 2.8g; Fiber 2.9g; Sodium 440mg; Iron 4.24mg; Phosphorus 283mg; Vitamin $B_{12}$ 3.4mcg; Vitamin C 32.

**Duck with cherries and leek mashed potatoes:** Energy 616 cal; Protein 50.7g; Carbohydrate 64.4g of which sugars 32.8g; Fat 18.8 g of which saturates 5.2g; Fiber 7.8g; Sodium 400mg; Vitamin $B_1$ (thiamin) 0.4mg; Vitamin C 22.3mg.

**Egg, tomato, and onion roll:** Energy 300 cal; Protein 16.1g; Carbohydrate 43.3g of which sugars 6.6g; Fat 8.7g of which saturates 2.3g; Fiber 5.6g; Sodium 720mg; Calcium 234mg; Zinc 1.8mg; Folic acid 124mcg.

**Fruity oat bars:** (per 1/16 portion) Energy 200 cal; Protein 3.3g; Carbohydrate 25.8g of which sugars 15.6g; Fat 10.0g of which saturates 2.2g; Fiber 3.0g; Sodium 0g; Zinc 1.1mg; Iron 1.56 mg.

**Ginger and orange slaw:** Energy 60 cal; Protein 1.5g; Carbohydrate 13.9g of which sugars 13.5g; Fat 0.3g of which saturates 0g; Fiber 3.6g; Sodium 0g; Vitamin A 560mcg; Vitamin C 60mg.

**Gratin of potato:** Energy 196 cal; Protein 8.8g; Carbohydrate 28.9g of which sugars 4.4g; Fat 5.9g of which saturates 3.5g; Fiber 2.5g; Sodium 200mg; Calcium 190mg.

**Greek style tomato and white fish:** Energy 235 cal; Protein 25.2g; Carbohydrate 6.3g of which sugars 6.2g; Fat 12.3g of which saturates 1.9g; Fiber 2.7g; Sodium 100mg; Iodine 316mcg; Vitamin C 17.3mg; Vitamin $B_3$ (niacin) 4.5mg.

**Green beans and chorizo:** Energy 220 cal; Protein 10.6g; Carbohydrate 4.8g of which sugars 4.2g; Fat 17.7g of which saturates 5.7g; Fiber 3.4g; Sodium 40mg; Zinc 1.77mg; Vitamin C 15.5; Vitamin $B_1$ (thiamin) 0.37; Vitamin $B_{12}$ 1.0.

**Grilled sardine and cheese sandwich:** Energy 425 cal; Protein 29.5g; Carbohydrate 47.9g of which sugars 6.1g; Fat 14.0g of which saturates 4.6g; Fiber 4.7g; Sodium 840mg; Calcium 650 mg; Iron 3.7mg; Zinc 2.8mg; Vitamin $B_{12}$ 9.3 mcg; Vitamin D 3.0mcg.

**Herbed barley:** Energy 190 cal; Protein 5.7g; Carbohydrate 42.0g of which sugars 0.2g; Fat 1.1g of which saturates 0.1g; Fiber 8.0g; Sodium 200mg.

**Homemade fish sticks with piquant avocado dip:** Energy 370 cal; Protein 33.3g; Carbohydrate 13.3g of which sugars 2.8g; Fat 20.8g of which saturates 7.2g; Fiber 3.6g; Sodium 440mg; Calcium 185mg; Magnesium 68mg; Vitamin $B_2$ (riboflavin) 0.46mg; Vitamin $B_{12}$ 0.86mcg.

**Honey-roasted stone fruit:** Energy 112 cal; Protein 1.8g; Carbohydrate 27.7g of which sugars 27.7g; Fat 0.2g of which saturates 0g; Fiber 3.8g; Sodium 0g; Vitamin C 13.5g.

**Hot potato salad:** Energy 218 cal; Protein 2.9g; Carbohydrate 27.5g of which sugars 2.2g; Fat 11.6g of which saturates 1.7 ; Fiber 3.3g; Sodium 0g; Vitamin C 30.0mg.

**Hungarian goulash:** Energy 265 cal; Protein 28.6g; Carbohydrate 15.3g of which sugars 9.8 Fat 10.3g of which saturates 3.1g; Fiber 3.8g; Sodium 200mg; Zinc 7.2mg; Vitamin A 675 mcg.

**Italian chicken gnocchi:** Energy 465 cal; Protein 27.3g; Carbohydrate 72.0g of which sugars 11.3g; Fat 9.6g of which saturates 1.6g; Fiber 10.4g; Sodium 320mg; Iron 4.6mg; Vitamin C 28mg; Folate 90mcg.

**Jambalaya:** Energy 520 cal; Protein 35.7g; Carbohydrate 72.5g of which sugars 6.1g; Fat 11.7g of which saturates 4.2g; Fiber 3.2g; Sodium 1,000mg; Vitamin $B_1$ (thiamin) 0.4mg; Vitamin $B_3$ (niacin) 3.57mg; Vitamin $B_{12}$ 4.5mcg.

**Kachumbari:** Energy 23 cal; Protein 1.0g; Carbohydrate 4.3g of which sugars 3.8g; Fat 0.3g of which saturates 0.1g; Fiber 1.7g; Sodium 100mg; Vitamin C 41mg.

**Lamb and green pepper kabobs with tzatziki:** Energy 353 cal; Protein 29.1g; Carbohydrate 16.4g of which sugars 9.2g; Fat 19.6g of which saturates 7.2g; Fiber 3.7g; Sodium 320mg; Vitamin $B_{12}$ 2.0mcg; Vitamin C 50mg; Zinc 4.0mg.

**Mango and lime dessert:** Energy 150 cal; Protein 8.1g; Carbohydrate 21.8g of which sugars 21.0g; Fat 4.0g of which saturates 0.6g; Fiber 5.6g; Sodium 0g; Calcium 464mg; Vitamin A 175mcg; Vitamin C 57mg.

**Mediterranean vegetable packages:** Energy 270 cal; Protein 9.2g; Carbohydrate 26.6g of which sugars 5.5g; Fat 14.2g pf which saturates 4.2g; Fiber 1.9g; Sodium 560mg; Vitamin C 25 mg.

**Mexican brunch:** (analysis with whole wheatl tortilla). Energy 387 cal; Protein 18.9g; Carbohydrate 59.9g of which sugars 14.9g; Fat 10.0g of which saturates 2.6g; Fiber 9.4g; Sodium 280mg; Iron 4.5mg; Vitamin C 15.3mg; Folate 100mcg.

**Moroccan hummus with flatbread:** (with 1 whole wheat pita bread*). Energy 172 cal (376 cal*); Protein 5.9g(14.9g*); Carbohydrate 10.0g of which sugars 0.5g (49.3g of which sugars 3.0g*); Fat 12.4g of which saturates 1.7g (14.7g* of which saturates 2.1g*); Fiber 3.6g (7.8g*); Sodium 240g (280g*); Iron 4.0mg (27mg*); Zinc 2.46mg (35mg*).

**Moroccan lamb stew:** Energy 333 cal; Protein 25.4g; Carbohydrate 17.8g of which sugars 16.3g; Fat 18.7g of which saturates 7.8g; Fiber 4.5g; Sodium 80mg; Iron 4.2mg; Zinc 5.3 mg; Vitamin $B_{12}$ 2.33mcg.

**Mozzarella turkey with fig and ginger preserves:** Energy 278 cal; Protein 33.8g; Carbohydrate 7.1g of which sugars 6.6g; Fat 12.8g of which saturates 6.8g; Fiber 2.0g; Sodium 200mg; Calcium 190mg; Vitamin $B_3$ (niacin) 6.5mg; Vitamin $B_{12}$ 1.7mcg.

**Mushroom and asparagus omelet:** Energy 297 cal; Protein 21.6g; Carbohydrate 2.3g of which sugars 2.0g; Fat 23.2g of which saturates 4.7g; Fiber 3.1g; Sodium 200mg; Iron 3.7mg; Zinc 2.8mg; Vitamin D 2.5mcg; Folate 138mcg; Iodine 76mcg.

**Mushroom stuffed chicken with green lentils:** Energy 263 cal; Protein 30g; Carbohydrate 19.9g of which sugars 1.6g; Fat 7.6g pf which saturates 1.4g; Fiber 4.1g; Sodium 500mg; Iron 5.0mg; Copper 0.6mg; Zinc 3.00mg.

**Paella:** Energy 455 cal; Protein 33.4g; Carbohydrate 58.7g of which sugars 7.8g; Fat 9.1g of which saturates 1.4g; Fiber 6.2g; Sodium 400mg; Zinc 2.9mg; Vitamin C 45mg; Vitamin A 460mcg.

**Orange and mint couscous:** (based on regular [not whole-grain] couscous). Energy 142 cal; Protein 3.4g; Carbohydrate 32.5g of which sugars 6.6g; Fat 0.6g of which saturates 0g; Fiber 2.6g; Sodium 0g; Vitamin C 25.0mg.

**Orange and pomegranate salad:** Energy 115 cal; Protein 2.6g; Carbohydrate 27.3g of which sugars 27.1g; Fat 0.3 g of which saturates 0g; Fiber 4.1g; Sodium 0g; Folic acid 75mcg; Vitamin C 94mg.

**Orange bran muffins:** Energy 178 cal; Protein 3.9g; Carbohydrate 29.9g of which sugars 13.1g; Fat 5.6g pf which saturates 0.6g; Fiber 2.4g; Sodium 80mg.

**Pasta primavera:** Energy 435 cal; Protein 18.7g; Carbohydrate 67.6g of which sugars 6.1g; Fat 11.7g of which saturates 4.1g; Fiber 14.4g; Sodium 120mg; Iron 5.0mg; Vitamin C 25.1mg; Vitamin $B_3$ (niacin) 3.5mg.

**Patatas bravas:** Energy 236 cal; Protein 5.8g; Carbohydrate 35.6g of which sugars 7.3g; Fat 9.1g of which saturates 0.8g; Fiber 5.2g; Sodium 80mg; Vitamin $B_6$ 0.55mg; Vitamin A 218mcg; Vitamin C 22.7mg.

**Peanut satay sauce:** Energy 142 cal; Protein 5.5g; Carbohydrate 2.4g of which sugars 1.6g; Fat 12.4g of which saturates 3.4g; Fiber 1.6g; Sodium 300mg.

**Pears in chocolate sauce:** Energy 300 cal; Protein 2.8g; Carbohydrate 49.9g of which sugars 49.9g; Fat 11.4g of which saturates 7.0g; Fiber 5.0g; Sodium 0g

**Pork with pineapple:** Energy 357 cal; Protein 34.8g; Carbohydrate 29.1g of which sugars 27.1g; Fat 12.2g of which saturates 2.5g; Fiber 4.5g; Sodium 100mg; Vitamin $B_1$ (thiamin) 1.0mg; Vitamin $B_3$ (niacin) 6.9mg.

**Potato-topped creamy fish casserole:** Energy 406 cal; Protein 36g; Carbohydrate 44.5g of which sugars 8.5g; Fat 10.6g of which saturates 3.8g; Fiber 4.4g; Sodium 800mg; Calcium 233mg; Vitamin $B_3$ (niacin) 7.2mg; Magnesium 90mg.

**Pot roasted chicken:** Energy 513 cal; Protein 38.9g; Carbohydrate 34.4g of which sugars 9.4g; Fat 25.5g of which saturates 6.6g; Fiber 8.1g; Sodium 520mg; Vitamin $B_3$ (niacin) 7.18mg; Folate 119mcg; Zinc 2.84mg; Vitamin A 719mcg.

**Pot roasted lamb shanks:** Energy 340 cal; Protein 32.00g; Carbohydrate 19.5g of which sugars 11.2g; Fat 14.9g of which saturates 4.6g; Fiber 3.9g; Sodium 120mg; Iron 3.76mg; Zinc 4.94mg; Vitamin A 1,415 mcg; Vitamin $B_3$ (niacin) 3.7mg.

**Quinoa and sunflower seeds:** Energy 260 cal; Protein 9.9g; Carbohydrate 35.0g of which sugars 3.7g; Fat 10.0g of which saturates 1.2g; Fiber 0.9g; Sodium 120mg; Iron 5.2mg; Zinc 2.4mg; Vitamin E 3.2mg.

**Quinoa, feta, and spinach salad:** Energy 386 cal; Protein 18.9g; Carbohydrate 35.9g of which sugars 5.8g; Fat 19.5g of which saturates 7.3g; Fiber 1.5g; Sodium 800mg; Calcium 290mg; Iron 5.9mg; Zinc 2.8mg; Vitamin $B_3$ (niacin) 3.2mg; Vitamin C 20.0mg; Vitamin A 475mcg.

**Raisin and apple pancakes:** (2 pancakes and 1 tbsp 3% fat plain yogurt). Energy 410 cal; Protein 14.9g; Carbohydrate 71.3g of which sugars 26.9g; Fat 9.2 g of which saturates 2.4g; Fiber 6.2g; Sodium 120mg; Calcium 235mg; Magnesium 69mg; Zinc 2.45mg; Vitamin $B_3$ (niacin) 3.4mg.

**Raspberry and pomegranate gelatin:** (based on using xylitol and regular [not sugar-free] syrup). Energy 73 cal; Protein 3.3g; Carbohydrate 18.1g of which sugars 10.7g; Fat 0.2g of which saturates 0 g; Fiber 2.8g; Sodium 0 g; Vitamin C 38mg.

**Raspberry oatmeal with walnuts:** Energy 380 cal; Protein 14.8g; Carbohydrate 50.0g of which sugars 23.0g; Fat 14.9g of which saturates 4.0g; Fiber 6.8g; Sodium 80mg; Calcium 350mg; Vitamin $B_3$ (niacin) 3.4mg; Magnesium 96mg.

**Ratatouille with halloumi and bread:** Energy 450 cal; Protein 21.5g; Carbohydrate 42.6g of which sugars 10.2g; Fat 22.4g of which saturates 11.5g; Fiber 4.9g; Sodium 960mg; Vitamin C 45mg; Vitamin A 280mcg.

**Roasted baby vegetables with tofu:** (based on 3 portions). Energy 193 cal; Protein 10.6g; Carbohydrate 10.6g of which sugars 8.7g; Fat 12.3g of which saturates 1.7g; Fiber 4.5g; Sodium 120mg; Calcium 544mg; Vitamin C 46.

**Roasted beets and butternut squash:** Energy 136 cal; Protein 2.7g; Carbohydrate 15.6g of which sugars 11.2g; Fat 7.5g of which saturates 1.0g; Fiber 3.9g; Sodium trace; Folate 75mcg; Vitamin A 500mcg.

**Roasted pepper and olive bruschetta:** Energy 172 cal; Protein 3.1g; Carbohydrate 17.5g of which sugars 4.1g; Fat 10.5g of which saturates 1.7g; Fiber 2.9g; Sodium 1,000mg; Vitamin A 577mcg.

**Roasted pork balls and vegetables:** Energy 444 cal; Protein 24.7g; Carbohydrate 39.9g of which sugars 12.8g; Fat 21.8g of which saturates 5.4g; Fiber 5.5g; Sodium 160mg; Vitamin $B_1$ (thiamin) 0.8mg; Vitamin C 50mg; Vitamin A 900mcg.

**Roasted red pepper pâté:** Energy 200 cal; Protein 2.0g; Carbohydrate 7.4g of which sugars 6.5g; Fat 18.1g of which saturates 8.1g; Fiber 2.2g; Sodium 40mg; Vitamin A 575mcg; Vitamin C 62.2mg.

**Romaine, chicken and croutons:** Energy 390 cal; Protein 20.6g; Carbohydrate 28.4g of which sugars 6.0g; Fat 21.6g of which saturates 3.8g; Fiber 6.9g; Sodium 280mg; Vitamin $B_3$ (niacin) 7.9mg; Folate 75mcg; Vitamin C 70mg.

**Salmon and asparagus en croûte:** Energy 413 cal; Protein 25.8g; Carbohydrate 26.2g of which sugars 3.3g; Fat 22.7g of which saturates 3.4g; Fiber 1.5g; Sodium 320mg; Vitamin D 4.6mcg; Omega 3 3.9g.

**Sardine and red pepper strudels:** Energy 325 cal; Protein 17.5g; Carbohydrate 31.4g of which sugars 5.8g; Fat 14.5g of which saturates 2.2g; Fiber 1.9g; Sodium 500mg; Calcium 258mg; Vitamin C 30mg; Vitamin D 2.5mcg; Vitamin $B_{12}$ 7.5mg.

**Sardines with avocado and cherry tomatoes:** Energy 527 cal; Protein 24.0g; Carbohydrate 3.9g of which sugars 2.8g; Fat 46.0g of which saturates 8.3g; Fiber 4.6g; Sodium 200mg; Iodine 75mcg; Vitamin C 25mg; Omega 3 3.42g; Vitamin D 20mcg.

**Sausage and orzo stew:** Energy 585 cal; Protein 24.7g; Carbohydrate 67.8g of which sugars 14.4g; Fat 26.0g of which saturates 7.4g; Fiber 7.2g; Sodium 900mg; Iron 4.0 mg; Vitamin C 25mg; Vitamin A 811mcg.

**Sea bass with pomegranate salsa:** Energy 226 cal; Protein 27.1g; Carbohydrate 9.8g of which sugars 9.3g; Fat 9.0g of which saturates 1.4g; Fiber 1.8g; Sodium trace; Vitamin $B_3$ (niacin) 5.0mg; Calcium 186mg.

**Sesame and coriander chicken with mango salsa:** Energy 308 cal; Protein 36.3g; Carbohydrate 10.9g of which sugars 9.7g; Fat 14.6g of which saturates 2.8g; Fiber 5.6g; Sodium 160mg; Zinc 3.5mg; Vitamin C 59mg; Vitamin $B_3$ (niacin) 6.37mg; Vitamin $B_{12}$ 1.6mcg.

**Smoked mackerel, ricotta, and beet bruschetta:** Energy 209 cal; Protein 8.9g; Carbohydrate 15.9g of which sugars 2.6g; Fat 12.6g of which saturates 3.4g; Fiber 1.1g; Sodium 400mg; Iodine 38mcg; Vitamin D 1.72mcg; Vitamin $B_{12}$ 1.55mcg; Omega 3 1.4g.

**Smoked salmon flakes with herbed lentils:** Energy 305 cal; Protein 33.1g; Carbohydrate 23.6g of which sugars 2.7g; Fat 9.3g of which saturates 3.5g; Fiber 7.3g; Sodium 520mg; Iron 5.33mg; Omega 3 2.8g; Zinc 2.3mg; Vitamin D 3.7mcg estimated.

**Spicy green edamame:** Energy 111 cal; Protein 6.8g; Carbohydrate 7.0g of which sugars 1.4g; Fat 6.3g of which saturates 0.8g; Fiber 5.6g; Sodium 0g; Vitamin C 30mg.

**Spinach stuffed chicken breasts with prosciutto:** Energy 313 cal; Protein 40.2g; Carbohydrate 0.3g of which sugars 0.2g; Fat 17.0g of which saturates 6.8g; Fiber 1.0g; Sodium 280mg; Vitamin A 314mcg; Vitamin $B_3$ (niacin) 8.5mg.

**Spinach with dried currants and pine nuts:** Energy 240 cal; Protein 4.4g; Carbohydrate 18.2g of which sugars 18.1g; Fat 17.3g of which saturates 1.7g; Fiber 3.9g; Sodium trace; Vitamin A 770mcg; Vitamin E 3.6mg

**Steak and broccoli with noodles:** Energy 416 cal; Protein 35.4g; Carbohydrate 30.1g of which sugars 6.6g; Fat 17.7g of which saturates 3.2g; Fiber 5.7g; Sodium 520mg; Iron 4.2mg; Vitamin C 35mg; Vitamin $B_{12}$ 2.2mcg.

**Strawberry mousse:** Energy 127 cal; Protein 8.4g; Carbohydrate 24.2g of which sugars 24.2g; Fat 0.3g of which saturates 0.1g; Fiber 2.3g; Sodium 0g; Vitamin C 70mg.

**Stuffed portobello mushrooms:** Energy 325 cal; Protein 18.9g; Carbohydrate 22.3g of which sugars 1.7g; Fat 18.4g of which saturates 3.3g; Fiber 5.2g; Sodium 440mg; Calcium 313mg; Vitamin $B_2$ (riboflavin) 0.36mg; Vitamin $B_3$ (niacin) 3.73mg; Vitamin $B_{12}$ 0.39mcg.

**Summer fruit compote:** (values given for sugar; those for xylitol in parenthesis). Energy 147 cal (109); Protein 1.9g (1.9g) Carbohydrate 36.4g (35.2g) of which sugars 36.4g (10.2g; Fat 0.3g (0.3g) of which saturates 0g (0g); Fiber 10.4g (10.4g); Sodium 0g (0g); Vitamin C 62.2mg (62.2mg).

**Sweet potato and chestnut jalousie:** (based on ⅙ portion). Energy 556 cal; Protein 6.6g; Carbohydrate 64.7g of which sugars 13.7g; Fat 30.1g of which saturates 15.2g; Fiber 9.9g; Sodium 400mg; Vitamin A 1171mcg; Copper 0.65mg.

**Tabbouleh with pine nuts:** Energy 313 cal; Protein 8.3g; Carbohydrate 30g of which sugars 4.2g; Fat 18.3g of which saturates 2.2g; Fiber 6.8g; Sodium trace; Magnesium 12mg; Iron 4.5mg; Zinc 1.9mg; Vitamin C 19.6mg.

**Tarka dhal:** Energy 304 cal; Protein 18.9g; Carbohydrate 45.7g of which sugars 3.9g; Fat 7.0 g of which saturates 0.6g; Fiber 9.7g; Sodium 120mg; Iron 6.9mg; Zinc 2.5mg.

**Tarragon sauce:** Energy 61 cal; Protein 1.1g; Carbohydrate 2.4g of which sugars 1.0g; Fat 5.2g of which saturates 1.8g; Fiber 0.3g; Sodium 0g.

**Teriyaki turkey with sesame cucumber salad:** Energy 296 cal; Protein 13.1g; Carbohydrate 5.2g of which sugars 4.1g; Fat 15.6g of which saturates 1.6g; Fiber 2.0g; Sodium 600mg; Vitamin $B_3$ (niacin) 8.3mg; Vitamin E 2.6mg.

**Tomato, basil, and mozzarella bruschetta:** Energy 197 cal; Protein 7.5g; Carbohydrate 16.6g of which sugars 3.1g; Fat 11.7g of which saturates 4.7g; Fiber 2.0g; Sodium 240mg; Vitamin C 15.3mg.

**Traditional rice pudding:** Energy 158 cal; Protein 7.5g; Carbohydrate 28.1g of which sugars 9.4g; Fat 3.3g of which saturates 1.9g; Fiber 0.5g; Sodium 40mg; Calcium 228mg.

**Tuna and vegetable pasta casserole:** Energy 450 cal; Protein 32.4g; Carbohydrate 34.1g of which sugars 9.2g; Fat 21.8g of which saturates 7.1g; Fiber 4.0g; Sodium 400mg; Calcium 250mg; Vitamin C 50mg; Iodine 52mcg; Vitamin $B_{12}$ 3.6mcg.

**Tuna steaks with sun-dried tomato crust and lime dressing:** Energy 407 cal; Protein 45.4g; Carbohydrate 14.0g of which sugars 2.9g; Fat 19.3g of which saturates 5.1g; Fiber 1.9g; Sodium 200mg; Vitamin D 12.3mcg; Omega 3 2.24g.

**Turkey herb burgers with fruity salsa:** (48g whole wheat roll with olive spread, ⅓ recipe salsa, and 12 sprigs of watercress). Energy 343 cal; Protein 25.8g; Carbohydrate 31.8g of which sugars 10.4g; Fat 13.5g of which saturates 2.3g; Fiber 34.4g; Sodium 400mg; Zinc 2.86mg; Selenium 15mcg; Vitain $B_1$ (thiamin) 0.26mg; Vitamin $B_3$ (niacin) 6.25mg; Vitamin C 32.3mg.

**Two pear salad:** Energy 310 cal; Protein 2.2g; Carbohydrate 19.8g of which sugars 18.8g; Fat 25.5g of which saturates 4.1g; Fiber 6.5g; Sodium 0g; Vitamin E 3.9mg.

**Tzatziki with raw vegetables:** Energy 123 cal; Protein 9.4g; Carbohydrate 7.6g of which sugars 6.8g; Fat g 6.2g of which saturates 1.0g; Fiber 2.9g; Sodium 240mg; Vitamin A 181mcg; Folate 75mcg; Vitamin C 29mg.

**Vegetable crepes with red pepper sauce:** (based on 2 small crepes plus ¼ recipe of vegetables and sauce). Energy 489 cal; Protein 24.1g; Carbohydrate 48.9g of which sugars 14.6g; Fat 23.3g of which saturates 5.4g; Fiber 10.5g; Sodium 280mg; Calcium 420mg; Zinc 2.7mg; Vitamin A 1,050mcg; Vitamin C 45.7mg; Vitamin $B_6$ 0.53mg; Folate 100mcg.

**Water chestnut and cashew nut stir fry:** Energy 384 cal; Protein 12.2g; Carbohydrate 36.4g of which sugars 10.1g; Fat 21.1g of which saturates 3.3g; Fiber 6.8g; Sodium 240mg; Vitamin A 337mcg; Vitamin C 43.0mg; Iron 3.9mg.

**Watercress and salmon salad:** Energy 320 cal; Protein 25.6g; Carbohydrate 5.4g of which sugars 4.8g; Fat 21.7g of which saturates 7.7g; Fiber 1.6g; Sodium 200mg; Vitamin D 5.5mcg; Vitamin A 210mcg; Omega 3 2.7g.

**Wild mushroom and rosemary sauce:** Energy 59 cal; Protein 1.6g; Carbohydrate 3.6g of which sugars 0.3g; Fat 4.3g of which saturates 0.8g; Fiber 0.9g; Sodium 80mg.

**Wild rice pilaf with fish, peas, and capers:** Energy 448 cal; Protein 34.4g; Carbohydrate 63.2g of which sugars 3.3g; Fat 8.3g of which saturates 1.0g; Fiber 6.1g; Sodium 400mg; Zinc 3.5mg; Vitamin $B_3$ (niacin) 6.5mg ; Vitamin $B_{12}$ 1.25mcg.

# INDEX

## A

Activity 31
Alcohol 34
Almond rice 136
Apple and berry oat crisp 148
Apple, sage, and walnut sauce 104
Asparagus
    risotto 74
    steaming 80
Aversions 36
Avocado and cherry tomato salad 117

## B

Baba ganoush with bread and
    asparagus tips 56
Baked
    beef and sour cherries 100
    figs with pistachios and
        honey yogurt 146
Bake, recipes
    Carrot sheet cake 150
    Cheddar and sun-dried
        tomato biscuits 153
    Chocolate Brazil brownies
        152
    Fruity oat bars 149
    Orange bran muffins 151
Barley and roasted vegetable salad
    with pumpkin seeds 71
Bean and salsa wrap 68
Beef
    and beet sandwich 68
    in beer 93
Berry
    smoothie 40
    yogurt breakfast 53
Birth weight 9
Black
    beans 54
    eyed-pea, dried currant, and
        fresh mint stew 126
Blackberry sauce 104
Bouquet garni 107
Brazil nut burgers 129
Breakfast
    cereals 19
    recipes
        Berry yogurt breakfast 53
        Citrus salad bowl 51
        Mexican brunch 54
        Mushroom and asparagus
            omelet 55
        Raisin and apple

pancakes 52
Raspberry oatmeal with
    walnuts 51
working 40
Breastfeeding 41
Broccoli with almonds 133
Broiling 102
Brushettas 58
Butternut squash casserole with
    halloumi and pomegranate 123

## C

Caffeinated drinks 34, 35
Calcium 11
Calcium-rich
    alternatives 23
    recipes 22
Canola oil 150
Carbohydrates 10
Carrot sheet cake 150
Casserole of duck and shallots with
    peaches 84
Cheddar and sun-dried tomato
    biscuits 153
Cheese
    shredding 153
    safe choices 31
Cherries, pitting 88
Chicken marinade 103
Chicken recipes
    Chicken with pine nuts and
        prunes 85
    Chocolate and spicy chicken 86
    Mushroom stuffed chicken
        with green lentils 90
    Romaine, chicken, and
        croutons 72
    Sesame and coriander
        chicken with mango salsa 91
    Spinach stuffed chicken
        breasts with prosciutto 92
Chile heat 86
Chinese
    beef and noodles 75
    pork with plums 97
Chocolate
    and chilli chicken 86
    Brazil brownies 152
    brioche pudding 147
Chorizo and black-eyed peas with
    Israeli couscous 76
Citrus salad bowl 51
Constipation 37
Copper 13

Crab
    cakes with watercress and
        orange salad 111
    linguine 110
Cravings 36
Creamy vegetarian ground "beef"
    122
Crepes 125
Curly kale with garlic cherry
    tomatoes 132

## D

Dessert, recipes
    Apple and berry oat crisp 148
    Baked figs with pistachios
        and honey yogurt 146
    Chocolate brioche pudding 147
    Dried fruit salad 142
    Honey-roasted stone fruit 145
    Mango and lime dessert 143
    Orange and pomegranate
        salad 140
    Pears in chocolate sauce 144
    Raspberry and pomegranate
        gelatin 140
    Strawberry mousse 141
    Summer fruit compote 142
    Traditional rice pudding 145
Diet, high protein 31
Dip, recipes
    Baba ganoush 56
    Moroccan hummus 64
    Piquant avocado dip 66
    Tzatziki 63
Dried fruit salad 142
Duck
    legs 84
    nutrients 23
    recipes
        Casserole of duck and
            shallots with peaches 84
        Duck and Asian
            mushroom stir-fry 87
        Duck with cherries and leek
            mashed potatoes 88

## E

Eatwell plate 16
Egg, tomato, and onion roll 70
Eggs 24
    safety 32
Energy needs 30
Essential fatty acids 10

## F

Fats 10
Fatty foods 17
Fiber 10
    in breakfast cereals 19
First trimester
    menu plan 42
    needs 49
Fish 24
    recipes
        Easy ways with 24
        Greek style tomato and
            fish 112
        Homemade fish sticks
            with piquant avocado
            dip 66
        Potato-topped creamy
            fish casserole 113
        Salmon and asparagus en
            croûte 115
        Sardines with avocado
            and cherry tomatoes 117
        Sea bass with pomegranate
            salsa 114
        Smoked salmon flakes with
            herbed lentils 116
        Tuna and vegetable pasta
            casserole 118
        Tuna steaks with sun-dried
            tomato crust and lime
            dressing 119
    safety 32, 112
Flat fish, skinning 112
Folate 14, 27
Food
    groups 16
    preparation 33
Fruit coulis 142
Fruits 20
Fruity
    oat bars 149
    salsa 94

## G

Gestational diabetes 37
Ginger and orange slaw 131
Glycemic index 19
Grains 19
Gratin of potato 139
Greek style tomato and fish 112
Green
    beans and chorizo 57
    spicy edamame 135
Grilling 102

**H**
Heartburn 37
Herb marinade 103
Herbed barley 137
Herbs 22
Homemade fishsticks with piquant
    avocado dip 66
Honey 146
    -roasted stone fruit 145
Hot potato salad 138
Hungarian goulash 98
Hyperemesis gravidium 37

**I, J, K**
Iodine 13
Iron 12
Italian chicken gnocchi 81
Jambalaya 77
Kachumbari 130
Key nutrients 10

**L**
Lamb and pepper kabobs with
    tzatziki 109
Leek mashed potatoes 88
Legumes 24
Lime dressing 119
Little bites, snacks, and sandwiches
    Baba ganoush with bread and
        asparagus tips 56
    Barley and roasted vegetable
        salad with pumpkin seeds 71
    Bean and salsa wrap 68
    Beef and beet sandwich 68
    Egg, tomato, and onion roll 70
    Green beans and chorizo 57
    Grilled sardine and cheese
        sandwich 69
    Homemade fish sticks with
        piquant avocado dip 66
    Mediterranean vegetable
        packages 61
    Moroccan hummus with
        flatbread 64
    Patatas bravas 60
    Quinoa, feta, and spinach salad
        73
    Ratatouille with halloumi and
        bread 67
    Roasted pepper and olive
        bruschetta 59
    Roasted red pepper pâté 62
    Romaine, chicken, and croutons
        72

Sardine and red pepper strudels
    65
Smoked mackerel, ricotta, and
    beetr bruschetta 59
Tabbouleh with pine nuts 64
Tomato, basil, and mozzarella
    bruschetta 58
Tzatziki with raw vegetables 63
Watercress and salmon salad 73
Liver 33

**M**
Magnesium 12
Mango
    and lime dessert 143
    dicing 143
    salsa 91
Marinades 103
Marinated artichoke and tarragon
    stuffing 93
Meal plans 38
Meat recipes
    Baked beef and sour cherries
        100
    Beef in beer 93
    Chinese pork with plums 97
    Hungarian goulash 98
    Lamb and pepper kabobs with
        tzatziki 109
    Moroccan lamb stew 108
    Pork with pineapple 96
    Pot roasted lamb shanks 107
    Steak and broccoli with noodles
        101
Mediterranean vegetable packages
    61
Menu plans 38
Meringue 141
Mexican brunch 54
Milk and dairy foods 17, 22
Minerals 11
Moroccan
    hummus with flatbread 64
    lamb stew 108
Mozzarella turkey with fig and
    ginger preserves 89
Mushroom
    and asparagus omelet 55
    and onion stuffing 93
    -stuffed chicken with green
        lentils 90

**N**
Nausea 36
Newborn weeks
    menu plan 48
    needs 41
Niacin 14
Nuts and seeds 26, 32

**O**
Oily foods 27
One-pot dish recipes
    Asparagus risotto 74
    Chinese beef and noodles 75
    Chorizo and black-eyed peas
        with Israel couscous 76
    Italian chicken gnocchi 81
    Jambalaya 77
    Paella 82
    Pot roasted chicken 80
    Roasted pork and vegetables 78
    Sausage and orzo stew 79
    Wild rice pilaf with fish,
        peas, and capers 83
Orange
    and mint couscous 137
    and pomegranate salad 140
    bran muffins 151

**P**
Paella 82
Pan-frying 102
Paprika 98
Pasta primavera 123
Patatas bravas 60
Patés 32
Peanut satay sauce 106
Peanuts 27
Pears in chocolate sauce 144
Phyllo pastry 115
Pine nuts 134
Piquant avocado dip 66
Polychlorinated biphenyls (PCBs) 32
Pomegranate
    salsa 114
    substitutions 71
Pork
    roasted, and vegetables 78
    checking for doneness 96
    with pineapple 96
Potassium 11
Potatoes 19
Pot roasted
    chicken 80
    lamb shanks 107

Potato-topped creamy fish
    casserole 113
Prebiotics 23
Prepregnancy 9
Probiotics 23
Protein 10
Protein-rich foods 17

**Q, R**
Quinoa
    and sunflower seeds 138
    feta and spinach salad 73
Raisin and apple pancakes 52
Raspberries 51
Raspberry
    and pomegranate gelatin 140
    oatmeal with walnuts 51
Ratatouille with halloumi and bread
    67
Ready-to-eat meals 33
Red pepper sauce 125
Riboflavin 14
Rice, washing 83
Roasted
    baby vegetables with tofu 124
    beet and butternut squash 135
    pepper and olive bruschetta 59
    red pepper pâté 62
Romaine, chicken, and croutons 72

**S**
Safe food preparation 33
Salad recipes
    Avocado and cherry tomato
        117
    Barley and roasted vegetable
        with pumpkin seeds 71
    Citrus salad bowl 51
    Dried 142
    Ginger and orange slaw 131
    Hot potato 138
    Kachumbari 130
    Orange and pomegranate 140
    Quinoa, feta, and spinach 73
    Sesame cucumber 95
    Two pear 130
    Watercress and salmon 73
Salmon and asparagus en croûte
    115
Salsas
    fruity 94
    mango 91
    pomegranate 114
Salty foods 27

Sandwich recipes
  Bean and salsa wrap 68
  Beef and beet sandwich 68
  Egg, tomato, and onion roll 70
  Grilled sardine and cheese
    sandwich 69
  Roasted pepper and olive
    bruschetta 59
  Smoked mackerel, ricotta, and
    beet bruschetta 59
  Tomato, basil, and mozzarella
    bruschetta 58
Sardine
  and cheese sandwich, grilled 69
  and red pepper strudels 65
  with avocado and cherry
    tomatoes 117
Sauce recipes
  Apple, sage, and walnut 104
  Blackberry 104
  Peanut satay 106
  Red pepper 125
  Tarragon 105
  Wild mushroom and rosemary
    106
Sausage and orzo stew 79
Sauté pan 99
Sea bass with pomegranate salsa
  114
Seaweed 32
Second trimester
  menu plan 44
  needs 40
Seeds 32
Selenium 13
Sesame
  and coriander chicken with
    mango salsa 91
  cucumber salad 95
Shellfish recipes
  Crab cakes with watercress and
    orange salad 111
  Crab linguine 110
Shellfish
  nutrients 24
  safety 32
Sickness 36
Side dish recipes
  Almond rice 136
  Herbed barley 138
  Orange and mint couscous 137
  Quinoa and sunflower seeds 138
Smoked
  mackerel, ricotta, and beet
    bruschetta 59
  salmon flakes with herbed
    lentils 116
Sodium 11
Soy 24

Soy sauce, sodium reduced 95
Spinach
  -stuffed chicken breasts with
    prosciutto 92
  with dried currants and pine
    nuts 134
Starchy foods 17
Steak and broccoli with noodles
  101
Strawberry mousse 141
Stuffed portobello mushrooms 122
Stuffings 93
Sugary foods and drinks 17, 27
Summer fruit compote 142
Sun-dried tomato and cream
  cheese stuffing 93
Supplements 27
Sweet potato and chestnut jalousie
  127

T
Tabbouleh with pine nuts 64
Tarka dhal 128
Tarragon sauce 105
Teriyaki
  marinade 95
  turkey with sesame cucumber
    95
textured soy protein 27
Thiamin 13
Third trimester
  menu plan 46
  needs 40
Tomato, basil, and mozzarella
  bruschetta 58
Tomatoes, skinning 123
Traditional rice pudding 145
Tuna
  and vegetable pasta casserole
    118
  steaks with sun-dried tomato
    crust and lime dressing 119
Turkey recipes
  Mozzarella turkey with fig and
    ginger preserves 89
  Teriyaki turkey with sesame
    cucumber 95
  Turkey herb burgers with fruity
    salsa 94
Twins 9, 31
Two pear salad 130
Tzatziki with raw vegetables
  63

V
Vegetable
  nutrients 21
  pancakes with red pepper sauce
    125

recipes
  Broccoli with almonds 133
  Curly kale with garlic cherry
tomatoes 132
  Gratin of potato 139
  Ratatouille with halloumi
    and bread 67
  Roasted beet and butternut
    squash 135
  Roasted pepper and olive
    bruschetta 59
  Roasted red pepper pâté 62
  Spicy green edamame 135
  Spinach with dried currants
    and pine nuts 134
  Vegetable crepes with red
    pepper sauce 125
Vegetarian recipes
  Black-eye pea, dried currant,
    and fresh mint stew 126
  Brazil nut burgers 129
  Butternut squash casserole with
    halloumi and pomegranate
    121
  Creamy vegetarian ground
    "beef" 122
  Mediterranean vegetable
    packages 61
  Pasta primavera 123
  Roasted baby vegetables with
    tofu 124
  Stuffed portobello mushrooms
    122
  Sweet potato and chestnut
    jalousie 127
  Tarka dhal 128
  Vegetable crepes with red
    pepper sauce 125
  Water chestnut and cashew nut
    stir fry 128
Vitamin
  A 13
  $B_6$ 14
  $B_{12}$ 14
  C 14
  D 16

  E 16
  K 17
Vitamins 13

W, X, Y, Z
Walnut, prune, and cinnamon
  stuffing 93
Water 26
Water chestnut and cashew nut stir
  fry 128
Watercress and salmon salad 73
Weight 29
  gain 30
Wild
  mushroom and rosemary sauce
    106
  rice pilaf with fish, peas,
    and capers 83
Working breakfast 40
Zinc 13

## ACKNOWLEDGMENTS

*I'd like to acknowledge the work of Amy Carroll and Chrissie Lloyd who waited patiently as this book evolved. Also my family who have eaten every recipe in the book more than once, and who are my most reliable critics.*

index and acknowledgments